auditory

training

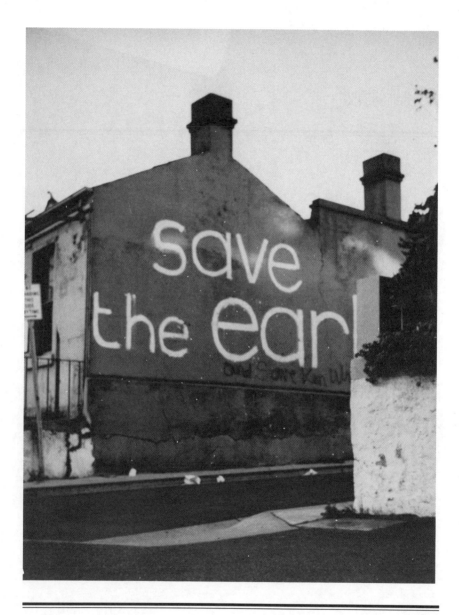

auditory training

norman p. erber

alexander graham bell
association for the deaf
3417 volta place, n.w.
washington, d.c. 20007

library of congress cataloging in publication data

auditory training
norman p. erber, ph.d.

library of congress catalogue card number 82–7820
isbn 0–88200–149–3
© 1982 by the a.g. bell association for the deaf
3417 volta place, n.w.
washington, d.c. 20007–2778

10 9 8 7 6 5 4 3 2

The purpose of this book is to help teachers, (re)habilitative audiologists, and parents of hearing-impaired children develop their skills as auditory instructors. My intent is not to promote a philosophy of oral/aural education or even to convince the reader that auditory learning is an important aspect of a hearing-impaired child's communicative development. Instead, I hope to provide sufficient background information and auditory instruction strategies to make a communication program as truly aural or "Total" as the instructor desires.

Unfortunately, in classes for the hearing impaired today, it is unusual for the auditory component of education to be given adequate emphasis. (Re)habilitative audiologists may direct considerable attention to the selection and maintenance of hearing aids, but rarely do they, teachers, or parents devote a comparable amount of time to helping the child learn to hear through the apparatus and thus through his impaired auditory system. In most instances, this situation has resulted from a lack of specific information, clear direction, or confidence in one's own auditory training abilities, rather than from a lack of interest or motivation.

Recently, it has become common practice for speech and hearing professionals to debate the relative merits of different types of amplification systems. A typical question might be, "What sort of electronic apparatus should we provide to these four children in the middle division of the school?" I often wonder whether this sort of question should be our basic concern. ("Without the right questions, there can be no right answers.") We probably would agree that the *quality* and *content* of the acoustic speech stimulus that is delivered to the child's ear(s) through his or her hearing aid(s) are considerably more important than *how many* aids the child wears, *where* the child carries them, or *whether* they are wired or wireless.

The material presented in this book will help the reader apply auditory training principles, regardless of the type of amplification apparatus preferred. The text provides some basic information regarding the speech perception abilities of hearing-impaired children, proposes a framework for establishing an auditory evaluation and training program, and then suggests numerous methods for providing hearing-impaired children with useful listening experiences. Practical suggestions are given on how to make auditory training "successful," that is, what to expect, how to demonstrate to the child and also to *oneself* that learning is occurring, and how to stay interested and motivated to continue helping the child learn. This approach to auditory training is presented in a straightforward and nontechnical way. Knowledge of audiology, speech acoustics, room acoustics, perception, learning principles, linguistics, or electronics is not required. However, a little knowledge in each of these areas can certainly make it easier for the reader to reach his or her goal. Nevertheless, I have risked a "cookbook" image and have provided numerous specific examples of auditory training activities because I believe this method of presentation can be useful in the initial stages of learning how to perform any task—baking an apple pie, or applying auditory training principles.

The ideas, methods, and materials described in these pages are based on my laboratory experiences at the Central Institute for the Deaf (St. Louis, Missouri) from 1970 to 1980, as a Research Associate, and also on my classroom experiences at the Glendonald School for Deaf Children (Kew, Victoria, Australia) during May through August, 1980, as Consultant in Educational Audiology. It was during the early years that I developed an understanding of the sensory capabilities of hearing-impaired children. Later, in Australia, I learned how this information could be applied in a practical manner by creative teachers to help hearing-impaired children develop their auditory abilities. I express my thanks to all of the people who have contributed directly or indirectly to the development of these concepts, especially the many hearing-impaired children whose auditory experiences I have shared.

Specifically, I would like to thank the following people, without whose help this text could not have evolved: Jenny Dowell and Geoff Plant, for their help in developing the GASP!; Gwen Rosengren, for her encouragement and support; Carol L. DeFilippo, Elizabeth Hightower, and S. Richard Silverman, for reading early versions of the manuscript and providing editorial assistance; Sheryl Hogg and Mary Saggau, for providing organizational help; Debbie Hunter and Ken Nicolai, for assisting in the preparation of illustrations; and Mary M. Sicking, for typing the numerous drafts of the manuscript. Preparation of the manuscript was supported by Program Project Grant NS 03856 from the National Institute of Neurological and Communicative Disorders and Stroke to the Central Institute for the Deaf.

Norman P. Erber
Lecturer in Rehabilitative Audiology
Department of Communication Disorders
Lincoln Institute of Health Sciences
625 Swanston Street
Carlton, Victoria, 3053, Australia

contents

historical background

auditory training

We may describe "auditory training" as the creation of special communication conditions in which teachers and others help hearing-impaired* children acquire many of the auditory speech-perception abilities that normally hearing children acquire naturally without their intervention. To many educators of the hearing impaired, applied auditory training consists of obtaining audiometric information, providing appropriate hearing aids, maintaining the amplification apparatus in good condition, and communicating through speech (audiovisually) with the child at all times. Many hearing-impaired children have quickly developed aural communication skills when parents and teachers did no more than modify the listening/learning environment in just these few ways. As a result, the children's auditory-visual perception of speech and acoustic monitoring of their own speech production improved.

In many cases, however, it has not been as easy to reach these communication goals. Instead, sustained progress has required the persistent efforts of teachers, audiologists, and parents who provide *auditory training*

---

*The term *hearing impaired* is used in this text in a general way to denote a deficiency in auditory perception (congenital or acquired) that is serious enough to interfere with normal development or maintenance of speech communication skills.

to the child, not only incidentally, but consciously on a carefully regulated basis. They created listening conditions in which visible cues (for lipreading) were intentionally minimized, and they helped the child develop auditory abilities beyond what the child might have achieved without such directed attention.

This chapter will review some of the work in auditory training of those educators who have made major contributions to the present state of the art. The purpose is to indicate the source of many of the ideas currently expressed by practitioners of auditory training and also to provide basic references the reader can consult for background information. This brief historical review will be presented in approximately chronological order.

robert gault

In the 1920s and 30s, Robert Gault and his colleagues, psychologists at Northwestern University (Evanston, Illinois), developed a simple vibrotactile aid for profoundly deaf people. This device allowed the deaf observers to acquire information about speech patterns conveyed by the temporal variations in the intensity of an utterance. During these decades, Gault and his coworkers collected considerable information about the sensory capabilities and limitations of the skin as a speech receptor. Numerous long-term training studies demonstrated that many hours of practice in receiving speech through vibrotactile transducers could enable a person to make increasingly finer distinctions among speech patterns (Gault, 1926b). This work was moderately successful, with many deaf observers learning to distinguish sentences in limited sets (Gault, 1926a), locate stress in words and sentences (Gault, 1930), and even identify or classify individual speech sounds (vowels and consonants) (Gault, 1926c; 1927; Weichbrodt, 1932).

Gault's goal was to describe the sensory capabilities of the skin with regard to speech-pattern information. His work firmly established the notion that even the minimal intensity-pattern cues available through a simple vibrotactile aid could benefit profoundly deaf lipreaders. They typically performed about 10 to 15% better on word identification tasks when they lipread with the vibrotactile device than when they used lipreading alone (Gault, 1928b). This finding has been confirmed more recently by many other researchers (Erber, 1972b). Gault's early work led to the development of multiple-vibrator aids (Gault, 1928a; Kringlebotn, 1968, Pickett & Pickett, 1963), an approach recently reestablished by several present-day researchers (see reviews by DeFilippo, 1979; Kirman, 1973).

max goldstein

In the 1930s and 40s, Max Goldstein, the founder of Central Institute for the Deaf (St. Louis, Missouri), popularized the "Acoustic Method," an approach to auditory training derived from the pioneering efforts of Victor Urbant-schitsch (1895) in Austria. In the 1890s, Urbantschitsch practiced systematic auditory training with congenitally hearing-impaired children demonstrating that children who appeared unresponsive to sound when first tested could improve their auditory performance after a period of concentrated instruction and practice. Thus, many pupils were able to progress from differentiation of vowels only, to perception of complete sentences. Goldstein was so impressed by this work in Europe that he introduced similar auditory training in the United States.

In his book and published manuscripts, Goldstein stressed the need for daily stimulation of the hearing-impaired child's remaining auditory sensitivity, and suggested numerous speech-pattern perception activities for this work (Goldstein, 1933, 1939). He emphasized that all children, regardless of the severity of the hearing loss, could benefit from experience in perceiving acoustic cues for speech. He also described the importance of audition in speech monitoring and control, as well as in speech reception. Goldstein developed both analytical and natural speech-perception exercises, which progress from perception of clearly audible vowels, through syllable drills, to identification of words and sentences. He proposed methods to effectively use the numerous sound and vibration conductors/transducers available at the time (for example, the Simplex tube (Figure 1–1), inflated balloons, and a covered megaphone), and strongly advocated the use of the first electrical hearing aids in auditory training (Figure 1–2). A considerable amount of his energy was devoted to convincing the *medical* profession of the auditory potential of hearing-impaired children, especially the role that hearing could play in their speech development.

clarence v. hudgins

In the 1940s and 50s, Clarence Hudgins at the Clarke School for the Deaf (Northampton, Massachusetts) carried out research studies with one of the first practical wired systems that offered group amplification (Hudgins, 1948, 1954). Through word identification testing, he demonstrated that regardless of the degree of their hearing loss hearing-impaired children could benefit from listening to speech at appropriately high acoustic levels. His data, collected over many years, indicated that listening practice could increase understanding through auditory perception, as well as improve speech and academic development. Hudgins also confirmed Gault's notion that even profoundly deaf children could learn to use the amplified patterns of speech to aid lipreading (Hudgins, 1954). All of these findings encouraged other educators to consider group amplification for their classrooms. Moreover, the research results served to raise their expectations for successful speech communication in their hearing-impaired pupils.

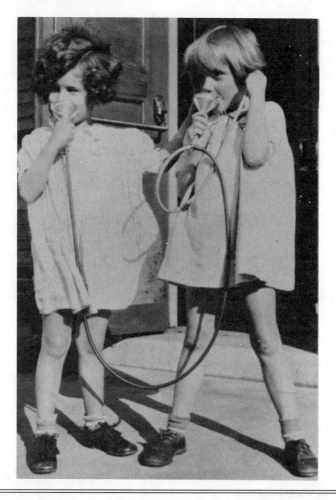

figure 1–1. Two hearing-impaired children use a Simplex Ear Tube to communicate through the sounds of speech (ca. 1935). The child on the right is able to hear her own voice as well as that of her friend.

auditory global method

In the 1950s and 60s, the "Auditory Global Method" was developed, applied, and promoted by Wedenberg (1951, 1954), Huizing (1959), Ewing and Ewing (1961), Whetnall and Fry (1964), van Uden (1970), and Simmons (1971) (see Calvert & Silverman, 1975). This approach to the use of a child's hearing capacity combines aided listening and lipreading. These educators strongly advocated early detection of hearing loss through the use of behavioral and electrophysiological methods, (for example, auditory evoked responses), so that appropriate hearing aids might be provided early in a child's life. The

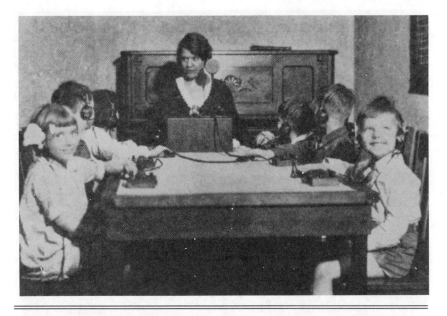

figure 1–2. A teacher and her pupils use an early electrical group hearing aid, the Acouvox. Acoustic input from a microphone is amplified and delivered through earphones at each pupil's station. The acoustic output level is adjusted for each child independently. The children also receive the output of the Acouvox through "teletactors" (vibrotactile transducers), which they feel with their fingertips (from Goldstein, 1939).

use of carefully selected hearing aids was considered a major factor in the aural habilitation of the hearing-impaired child. Other critical factors were involvement by the parents in their child's habilitation and their determination to provide useful speech and language stimulation. The Auditory Global Method represented a departure from the earlier acoustic methods in two respects. First, the pupils were encouraged to look as well as listen most of the time. Second, the method was based on a natural development of speech and language skills rather than the more analytical procedures employed by earlier educators such as Goldstein.

electronics industry

In the 1960s and 70s, a rapidly expanding electronics industry led to the successful miniaturization of hearing aid microphones and circuitry. Reliable behind-the-ear hearing aids were developed for children (Figure 1–3). Interest also turned to the creation and application of special amplification devices. Thus, for example, educators devoted increased attention to the low-fre-

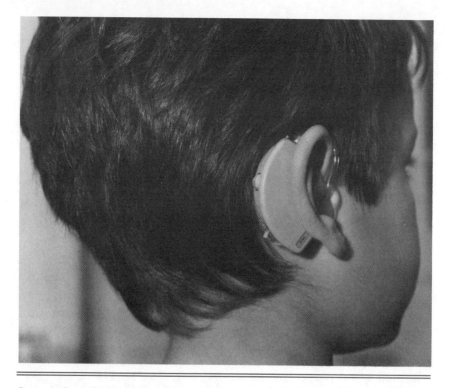

figure 1–3. A "behind-the-ear" hearing aid. Amplified sound is delivered to the child's ear through a small plastic tube and an earmold.

quency sensitivity of hearing-impaired children in order to provide amplified acoustic information in that frequency range (Asp, 1973). Ling (1964), Guberina (1964), and Briskey and Sinclair (1966) reported positive results in speech perception and production by extending effective amplification of hearing aids into the low frequencies. Others obtained equivocal results, perhaps due to amplification of unwanted background noise or to the likelihood of upward spread of masking (reduction in clarity) from intense low-frequency speech cues (Danaher & Pickett, 1975). Wideband (extended low-frequency) amplification also was introduced as one of several aspects of the Verbotonal system (Guberina, 1964). Proponents of this comprehensive method employed selective amplificaton in "optimal" frequency regions, vibrotactile aids, rhythmic speech instruction, and attention to intonation and stress patterns in developing the receptive and expressive language of young severely and profoundly hearing-impaired children. The importance of concentrated *individual* work with children also was strongly emphasized as an important factor contributing to success.

Other devices were designed to incorporate elaborate processing of the amplified speech signal. For example, Johannsen (1966) introduced the

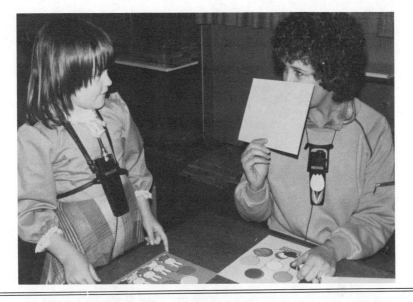

figure 1—4. A teacher uses a wireless FM transmission/amplification system to communicate with the hearing-impaired children in her classroom.

Transposer hearing aid, which electronically shifted high-frequency speech energy to a much lower frequency range. Others developed similar frequency shifting devices (Guttman & Nelson, 1968; Ling, 1968). With this sort of special apparatus, some profoundly deaf children could learn to detect high-frequency consonants with confidence (for example, / s, ʃ, f, θ /), and also to produce these speech sounds with greater consistency.

In the 1970s, designers directed considerable attention to increasing the amplification system's portability and developed high quality behind-the-ear hearing aids, usually worn binaurally. Manufacturers also introduced several types of wireless amplification systems that employed magnetic induction loops, radio-frequency transmission, or infrared radiation to convey speech energy (Ross & Tomassetti, 1980) (Figure 1—4). These special devices allowed the communicators greater mobility and thus encouraged more natural interaction between teacher and children. Furthermore, with these developments, it was possible to achieve high fidelity and relatively noise-free communication outside of an acoustically controlled classroom.

unisensory instruction

Instructional emphasis also shifted in the 1970's. Unisensory ("acoupedic") instruction as advocated by Beebe, (1953), Pollack (1970), and Grammatico (1974) gained popularity. The "acoupedic" program, so named by Huizing (1959) to differentiate it from other methods used at traditional preschools

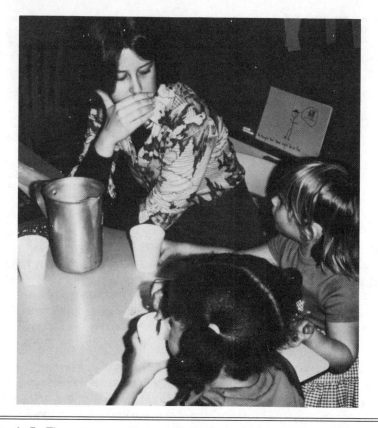

figure 1–5. The unisensory ("acoupedic") approach is used during a classroom activity.

for the deaf, is designed to help children reach their potential as *aural* communicators. The teacher/parent provides both carefully planned lessons and natural communication, but without allowing clear visibility of the talker's mouth. That is, the mouth is covered much of the time and lipreading is discouraged (Figure 1–5). Hence, concentrated individual instruction is strongly recommended rather than group work (as in a classroom) for this intense auditory practice. When the talker covers the mouth with a hand or a card, the child must develop his or her listening skills, and is encouraged to develop auditory vocabulary, auditory language competence, and an acoustic speech-feedback mechanism. One of the program's major goals is full early integration into regular classrooms. For a child with impaired hearing, a classroom of nonauditory communicators is considered detrimental to rapid development of an acoustically based language system. Nevertheless, many observers have suggested that an auditory-only approach cannot be used successfully with all children, especially those with extremely poor hearing. This remains a controversial issue.

the future

Recently, there has been great interest in the development of sophisticated hearing aid selection procedures (Pascoe, 1975; Skinner, 1980) and creation of superior earmolds (Fifield, Earnshaw, & Smither, 1980; Killian, 1981). Also, elaborate signal processing has been employed in newly designed hearing aid circuitry to compress or shift the speech signal into the limited hearing range of the impaired listener (Braida, Durlach, Lippmann, Hicks, Rabinowitz, & Reed, 1979; Villchur, 1978; Yanick & Freifield, 1978). At the same time, a renewed interest in nonauditory devices for the profoundly deaf has resulted in a return to the vibrotactile device as an important aid in auditory training (Asp, 1973; Erber, 1978; Schulte, 1978). Surgeons now can perform implantation of cochlear prostheses that electrically stimulate the auditory nerve (Clark, Pyman, & Bailey, 1979; House, 1976). It is not clear at present whether these surgical procedures provide significantly greater help to the profoundly deaf child than do less drastic approaches, such as the use of powerful hearing aids or vibrators (Martin, Tong, & Clark, 1981; Owens & Telleen, 1981).

summary

From the numerous developments of the past 50 years, one may conclude that carefully directed listening practice is a valuable experience for a hearing-impaired child, exerting a major positive influence on his or her communicative development. This has been recognized even by those clinicians and researchers who emphasize the amplification system itself as the primary rehabilitative tool. They now acknowledge that the young listener needs to *learn* how to interpret the sounds perceived through the electronic apparatus he or she carries. Consequently, very few teachers or educational audiologists now need to be convinced of the value of auditory training (or at least the provision of specialized listening practice); but many are unsure of how to proceed in an organized manner. Therefore, for teachers to provide auditory training with ease and efficiency, the training process itself must enable them to not only give their pupils confidence as successful listeners, but also to acquire confidence in their abilities as hearing therapists. The future demands a more unified, coherent approach to providing auditory learning experiences to hearing-impaired children.

speech
perception

This chapter will survey speech perception ability in hearing-impaired children, and examine how it relates to the ease with which they develop speech and oral language. We will review the capabilities and limitations of the various senses for speech perception, and we will briefly consider various speech-feedback devices, such as visual displays, hearing aids, and vibrotactile devices, that can be used to help a hearing-impaired child compensate for perceptual limitations. Teaching techniques that rely on a sequence of demonstration, perception, and imitation will be discussed with regard to their use in development of speech perception and speech production abilities.

speech perception and speech intelligibility

Figure 2–1a describes a general relation between the speech intelligibility of a group of hearing-impaired children and their hearing threshold levels for pure tones (Boothroyd, 1976). Speech intelligibility tends to be generally high (nearly 100% for the experienced listeners in this study) for children with hearing levels better than about 70 dB, but becomes progressively lower for children with poorer pure-tone thresholds. These lower levels of performance for severely and profoundly hearing-impaired children have been reported

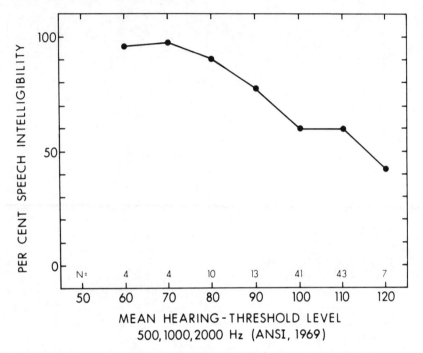

figure 2–1a. Acoustic speech intelligibility of 122 hearing-impaired children as a function of mean hearing level for 500-1000-2000 Hz in the better ear. Scores represent percentage of syllables correctly recognized by a group of normally hearing listeners from a set of sentences spoken by the children (from Boothroyd, 1976).

in several other studies as well (Monsen, 1978; Smith, 1975). They tend to parallel data depicting auditory speech-feature recognition by similar groups of hearing-impaired children (Figure 2–1b). The implication is that a child's ability to produce intelligible speech is related in a general way to his ability to perceive its spectral (pitch) and prosodic (pattern) qualities, although we know that many hearing-impaired children learn to produce numerous speech qualities they cannot hear (Smith, 1971).

It is acknowledged that most moderately, severely, and profoundly hearing-impaired children depend to a considerable extent on their vision for oral language learning and for speech communication. Lipreading plays a major role in speech perception and also a part in certain aspects of speech learning, as in attention to a teacher's articulatory pattern (Jenson, 1971). Accordingly, the possibilties and limitations of lipreading as a speech perception and feedback mode will be discussed. Then we will examine ways in which perception of acoustic cues from a hearing aid during auditory training can benefit a hearing-impaired child.

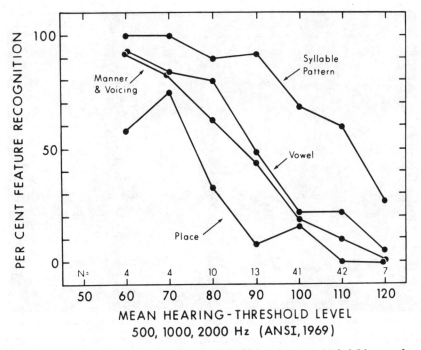

figure 2—1b. Group mean scores obtained by 122 hearing-impaired children on four acoustic speech-feature perception tests, shown as a function of mean hearing level for 500-1000-2000 Hz (from Boothroyd, 1976).

visual perception

visemes and speech communication

Typically, hearing-impaired children are unable to perceive all of the sounds of speech accurately through aided hearing and so substitute visual perception of articulation for the auditory perception of certain phonemes. The linguistic symbols they seem to use in lipreading are the visually observable positions* of the lips, teeth, tongue, and the surrounding facial surfaces. However, visual perception of an articulatory position alone usually is insufficient for the accurate identification of a speech element. For example, a closure of the lips, considered by itself, has no linguistic value; it even may signal an absence of communication (rest). But if a child perceives lip closure

---

* Although transition *movements*, as well as articulatory *positions*, are important for visual perception of speech, these dynamic events generally are not incorporated into theoretical analysis of visible speech features, at least at the present time.

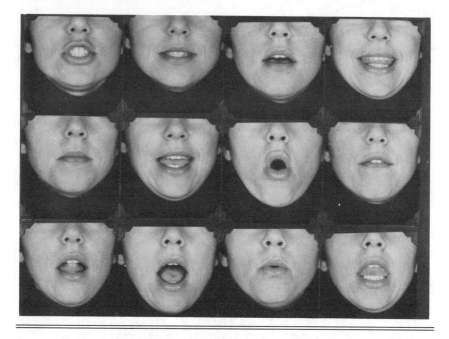

figure 2–2. Some articulatory positions (visemes) which according to theory form the basis for visual perception of speech through lipreading.

in combination with a subsequent lip opening, then this lip position becomes a visible marker of an articulatory gesture which corresponds to a particular set of phonemes in English (/ p, b, m /) (Figure 2–2).

The visually observable units of speech articulation have come to be called "visemes" (that is, homophenes, clusters) (Fisher, 1968). These visemes can convey linguistic information in a way similar to the phonemes of a language. Most speakers, however, do not consciously create visemes as they talk, but instead speak to generate *acoustically* correct sounds rather than *visually* distinguishable ones. Thus, visemes are unconscious visible byproducts of acoustic speech production. Nevertheless, although most hearing people are not aware of visemes, hearing-impaired children can learn to apply them as useful linguistic symbols (see Alich, 1967; DeFilippo, 1982).

Unfortunately, visemes are less efficient language symbols than are phonemes (speech sounds) or graphemes (printed letters) for several reasons: 1) numerous speech sounds are produced by similar, visible speech articulations (for example, / f, v /); 2) some speech gestures occur deep within the oral cavity and are not easily visible to the lipreader (for example, phonation (voice production), velar lowering (or nasal emission); and 3) coarticulation influences the visibility of many speech articulations; some visemes which can be identified in isolation become indistinguishable in combination.

For example, in the word *needles*, the phonetic elements / d /, / l /, and / z / blend to form one viseme. (Although one might argue that *all* of the articulatory configurations in this difficult word are perceived by the lipreader as a single viseme.)

In this way, approximately 40 English phonemes are reduced to about 9 to 14 visemes in conversational speech (Jeffers & Barley, 1971). In general, these visemes correspond to consonants that are confused with one another because certain speech features, such as voicing and nasality, are not visually apparent (for example, / t, d, n /) and to vowels commonly confused because of similarities in degree of lip spreading or rounding (for example, / I, ε / and / U, u /). The resulting ambiguities in this optical code would require the young hearing-impaired child to learn about our 40-phoneme spoken language system through a sensory channel that transmits considerably fewer than that number, if he or she were to learn through lipreading alone.

information available through lipreading

In spite of this apparent obstacle to communication, many hearing-impaired children do learn speech and language mainly through lipreading—assisted by useful acoustic cues from a hearing aid, natural gestures, written material, and help from a teacher.

consonants

Most lipreaders can distinguish consonants categorically on the basis of their points of articulation (for example, labial, alveolar, velar), although consonant recognition is affected by vowel context (Erber, 1971b, 1974b; Pesonen, 1968) (Figure 2–3). The consonants that children confuse visually with one another generally are those that differ instead on the basis of voicing or manner (rather than place) of articulation (Erber, 1972a). Apparently, even inexperienced lipreaders can learn to distinguish reliably among the places of consonant articulation (Erber, 1972a), and little specific practice seems required to reach this level of competence (Walden, Prosek, Montgomery, Sherr, & Jones, 1977). However, accurate identification of consonant visemes requires good optical conditions (Erber, 1971b, 1974a).

vowels

Lipreaders seem to vary in ability to accurately identify vowels, although they have little difficulty distinguishing between spread (front) and rounded (back) categories; these two types of lip pattern form very distinct visemes. Rather, it is more common for children to misidentify vowels produced in neighboring articulatory (lipshape) positions (Figure 2–4). Vowel identifica-

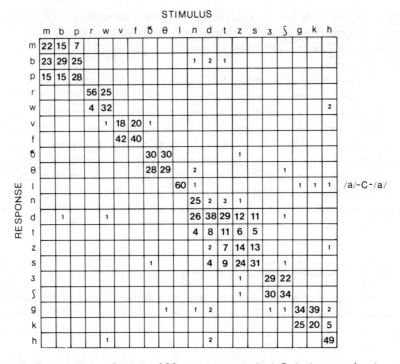

figure 2–3. Visual identification of 20 consonants in / ɑ / -C- / ɑ / context by six profoundly hearing-impaired children. Results are given in the form of a confusion matrix. Stimuli were presented under conditions of frontal illumination by a talker who articulated carefully (Erber, 1974b).

tion is relatively unaffected by distance, light level, or optical clarity (Erber, 1971b, 1974a). Although some vowel articulations may appear ambiguous, children usually can categorize gross mouth shapes correctly even under extremely poor optical conditions (Erber, 1979b).

words

Children usually can visually identify longer words, such as spondees (*football*), much more easily than shorter words, such as monosyllables (*cat*) (Erber, 1971b, 1974a). Two-syllable words with either iambic (*giraffe*) or trochaic (*father*) stress are intermediate in intelligibility. It seems that if more (stressed) syllables are in a word, then more visible cues are available to the child for identification. Experience suggests that a very important factor contributing to a word's visual intelligibility is the uniqueness of its visible articulatory pattern—the extent to which the word looks different from other words in the language (Argila, 1978).

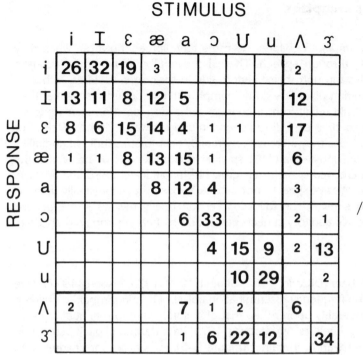

figure 2–4. Visual identification of 10 vowels in / b / -V- / b / context by five profoundly hearing-impaired children. Results are given in the form of a confusion matrix. Stimuli were presented under conditions of frontal illumination by a talker who articulated carefully.

sentences

Children are able to lipread short, syntactically simple sentences more easily than long, complex sentences (Clouser, 1976). Complicated syntactic transformations, such as embedded clauses, passive verb constructions, negatives, multiple subjects or objects, question forms, or various combinations of these make sentences more difficult to lipread (Schwartz & Black, 1967). Many hearing-impaired children seem to have the least difficulty with the subject-verb-object (-prepositional phrase) sentence frame, probably because this is a basic construction and is introduced early in their education.

A major problem in lipreading is that the coarticulation of speech elements in sentences often makes it difficult for the lipreader to specify word boundaries, especially where reduced syllable stress affects the clarity of articulation. To optimize comprehension of sentences, the lipreader must not only rely on vision for perception of speech rhythm and word emphasis, but also refer to linguistic memory for probable word sequences.

auditory perception

Most hearing-impaired children do more than lipread, however, when they communicate through speech. They also carefully *listen*—to the acoustic cues that pass through their hearing aids to their ears. Children with sensorineural hearing disorders do not simply perceive sounds as weaker than normal, as would result from a conductive hearing loss (for example, otitis media). Instead, their ears *distort* sound in unusual ways (Plomp, 1978). For example, loudness may increase very rapidly near the threshold of audibility, so that if a previously inaudible speaker now raises his or her voice, the loudness of perceived speech may grow disproportionately. Also, the normally distinctive qualities of speech may be changed, so that acoustically different words sound similar. The following section briefly reviews some general characteristics of auditory speech perception by hearing-impaired children.

voice pitch

Researchers (DiCarlo, 1962; Gengel, 1969, 1973; Risberg, 1977) have shown that the frequency discrimination ability of hearing-impaired children often is considerably poorer than that of children with normal auditory sensitivity. Risberg, Agelfors, and Boberg (1975) have described pitch perception abilities in the hearing impaired (Figure 2–5). In general, for children with hearing levels ranging from about 30 to 60 dB ("mild to moderate" loss), the ability to distinguish low frequencies (125 to 1000 Hz) is essentially unimpaired, that is, only about a 1 to 2 percent difference (in Hz) is required to hear the difference between two neighboring tones. For children with audiograms in the 70 to 90 dB hearing level (HL) range ("severe"), however, there are large individual differences in frequency discrimination, ranging from about 2 to 30 percent, that is, from nearly normal to moderately poor discrimination ability. For children with hearing thresholds poorer than about 100 dB HL ("profound" loss), frequency discrimination tends to be very poor; these children require a 5 to 40 percent difference in frequency to distinguish two tones. (This range of poor performance is comparable to that obtained vibrotactually from the hand, and may, in fact, reflect tactile responses from the ear.) A child's tone discrimination performance has been found to relate closely to his ability to recognize familiar words (Risberg, et al., 1975). Thus, it appears that the ability to distinguish nearby frequencies is an auditory skill basic to speech perception, and especially to identification of voice pitch and the formant spectra (concentrations of acoustic energy) of vowels and most consonants.

vowels

Many hearing-impaired children with moderate to severe hearing impairments seem unable to accurately perceive the frequency location of vowel

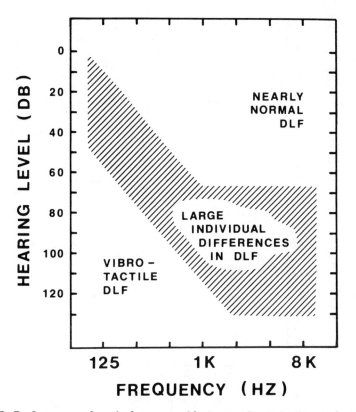

figure 2–5. Summary of results from several frequency discrimination studies. Three audiometric ranges were found to be associated with different degrees of DLF (difference limen for frequency). Large individual differences in DLF were obtained from children whose pure-tone thresholds were in the "severe" range (from Risberg et al., 1975).

formants, and so misidentify vowels produced in neighboring articulatory positions. For example, these children might identify the vowel / I / as / i / or / ε /, and thus might confuse the words *pin, team,* and *ten* (Figure 2–6). Other moderately to severely hearing-impaired children seem to have difficulty detecting the presence of the second (high) formant in vowels (Miller, 1956); consequently, they perceptually confuse "front" and "back" vowels that have similar first (low) formants, for example, / i / and / u /, as in *three* and *two* (Figure 2–6). When confronted with this perceptual ambiguity, some children will choose randomly between the two vowels (or words), while others will exhibit definite biases toward either the front or back vowel. Moreover, some severely hearing-impaired children exhibit both kinds of difficulty, they confuse vowels produced with similar articulation and also front/back pairs. A child with this complex type of auditory deficiency, when presented with the vowel / I /, may identify it as / i / or / ε /, or label it as / U / and thus identify

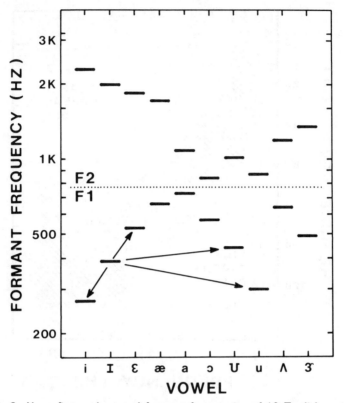

figure 2–6. Mean first and second formant frequencies of 10 English vowels, as produced by a group of adult males (Peterson & Barney, 1952). Arrows indicate formants similar in frequency to the first formant of the vowel / I /. These similarities may explain the tendency of some severely hearing-impaired children to confuse that vowel with the vowels / i, ε / and also with / ʊ, u / (Hack and Erber, 1982).

the word *pick* as *peek, pet,* or *put.* (Hack & Erber, 1982; Picket, Martin, Johnson, Smith, Daniel, Willis, & Otis, 1972; Smith, 1975). (Figure 2–6).

Test results indicate that even children with profound hearing impairments (those whose responses suggest that they perceive only intensity cues vibrotactually) can learn to distinguish between "strong" vowels (/ æ, a, , ʌ /) and those weaker in acoustic energy (/ i, I, ε, ʊ, u /), (Hack & Erber, 1982). Similar findings had been reported by Gault (1926c). Vowel classification simply on the basis of intensity cues, however, is much less precise in word or sentence context, where syllable stress can modify the relative intensities and durations.

consonants

Many of the consonant confusions experienced by moderately and severely hearing-impaired children are similar to those reported previously by Miller and Nicely (1955). In their study, normally hearing adults listened to consonants in syllabic context through electric filters or in noise backgrounds. Many researchers subsequently have used a basic filter analogy to describe or simulate hearing loss in a simple way (Boothroyd, 1967; Ross, Duffy, Cooker & Sargeant, 1973; Sher & Owens, 1974).

Listeners with moderate to severe hearing impairments typically have little difficulty distinguishing categorically among nasals, voiced stops, voiced fricatives, voiceless stops, and voiceless fricatives (Byers, 1973; Owens, Benedict & Schubert, 1972). That is, they tend to perceive these articulatory classes as separate from one another acoustically, but they confuse the consonants within each group. Our experience indicates that many children with more severe impairments often confuse voiced stops and fricatives with one another and similarly confuse their voiceless counterparts. Nevertheless, it appears that hearing-impaired children even with only minimal hearing usually can distinguish nasal and non-nasal consonants, although their precise labeling of / m / and / n / may be very poor (Erber, 1972a)(Figure 2–7). When nasal consonants are misclassified, they are most frequently confused with the liquids and semivowels / r, l, w, j / (Walden & Montgomery, 1975), which in turn may be confused with vowels having similar low-frequency

STIMULUS

	p	t	k	b	d	g	m	n
p	88	34	43	8	3	7	4	5
t	45	103	45	2	9	12	1	6
k	44	53	100	5	14	6	2	1
b	15	12	8	136	25	29	3	2
d	21	8	14	47	101	39	5	2
g	10	9	10	17	62	118		
m	2	2	3	5	4	4	147	95
n		4	2	5	7	10	63	114

RESPONSE

```
Severely hearing-impaired:
Auditory reception.
P(c)=50.38%   T(x;y)=1.06 bits
```

figure 2–7. Monaural auditory identification of 8 stop and nasal consonants in / a / -C- / a / context by five severely hearing-impaired children (Erber, 1972a).

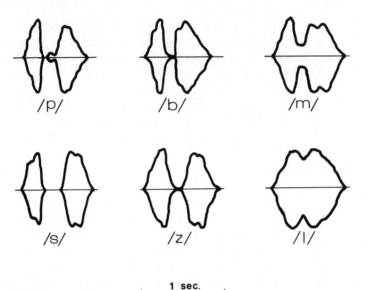

/p/   /b/   /m/

/s/   /z/   /l/

|⊢——— **1 sec.** ———⊣|

figure 2–8. Intensity patterns of six consonants spoken in the context / a / -C- / a /, as displayed on the screen of a storage oscilloscope. The amplitude and duration of intervocalic energy can provide information regarding the category of consonant that was presented (from Erber, 1978).

spectra. Consequently, words containing several consonants in the group / m, n, r, l, w, j / tend to be very difficult for severely hearing-impaired children to identify acoustically, especially when these phonemes appear in medial position (for example, *money, always, really, woman*).

Although the frequency discrimination abilities of most profoundly hearing-impaired children are poor, they usually can perceive changes in speech *intensity* as a function of time. Thus, for example, they are able to distinguish stop from voiced continuant consonants in a medial position, as the former class is characterized by a distinct break in the sound pattern and the latter is not (Figure 2–8). Initial or final stop consonants in words, however, may be labeled incorrectly. For example, in the word / kaet /, the energy bursts in / k / and / t / are weak and of relatively high frequency, and so produce little intensity disturbance before or after the vowel. Thus, a profoundly deaf child might not be able to distinguish between / kaet / and / ae / alone, because of a lack of high-frequency sensitivity.

Nasals and liquids/semivowels may be identified as a distinct consonant category (depending on speech context) on the basis of the slow rise and fall in intensity of the syllable pattern. And, so, many profoundly hearing-impaired children can learn to classify the pattern for / mæn / as different from / bæt), or as another example, the name *Bobby* from *Mommy*. To further illustrate the effect of the many intensity and duration cues occurring

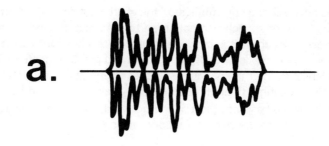

"THE BABY TOOK THE BROKEN
TOY TRAIN TO DADDY."

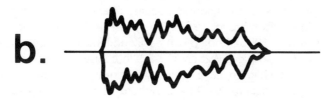

"THE LAMB ALWAYS RUNS AWAY
WHEN I MOVE MY HAND."

figure 2–9. Intensity patterns of two sample sentences: one contains mainly stop consonants (a); the other contains mainly continuant consonants (b). A profoundly hearing-impaired child can easily learn to distinguish contrastive patterns of this sort (from Erber, 1980b).

in connected speech, compare the patterns of the two sentences: "The baby took the broken toy train to daddy," and, "The lamb always runs away when I move my hand." (Figure 2–9). The first contains numerous stop consonants and thus brief silent intervals; the second does not.

    The general auditory capabilities and limitations of hearing-impaired children outlined above summarize the results of many research studies and clinical observations. These findings do not define a specific child's potential for auditory perceptual learning. The way in which a particular severely or profoundly hearing-impaired child learns to perceive and produce speech is complicated by the fact that he or she may hear many speech elements only after considerable spectral transformation (distortion) by hearing aids and ears. Some sounds of speech may not be audible at all. If the child is to succeed as an aural-oral communicator, the child must develop an effective, personal method for speech perception and for monitoring and controlling his or her own speech as it is produced. Often a teacher can help improve a child's speech-perception performance by giving practice in attending and assigning labels to the minimal acoustic cues (Bennett & Ling, 1977). The child can also be taught to apply strategies for making informed "guesses", when unsure, on the basis of typical phoneme, word, and sentence sequences. Both general activities are part of auditory training.

combined auditory-visual perception

Numerous studies have indicated that the *acoustic* speech-perception skills of *severely* hearing-impaired children differ considerably from those of children with *profound* hearing-impairments, especially regarding the ability to recognize the spectral qualities of speech components (Risberg, 1976). For instance, many severely hearing-impaired children can distinguish certain low-frequency vowel and consonant qualities nearly as well as can normally hearing children (Boothroyd, 1967; Erber, 1972a; Pickett & Martin, 1968; Pickett & Martony, 1970), and so can easily understand simple words such as numbers and spondees (Erber, 1974c). In contrast, because profoundly hearing-impaired children have difficulty discriminating sounds of neighboring frequency (Risberg, Agelfors, & Boberg, 1975), they generally are not good at distinguishing the spectral qualities of most vowels and consonants (Erber, 1972a; Boothroyd, 1976; Risberg, 1976); hence, they cannot identify even familiar words (Erber, 1974c, 1979d). In fact, profoundly hearing-impaired children seem to perceive little more than the overall intensity patterns of amplified acoustic speech signals through appropriately selected hearing aids (Erber, 1972b, 1979d; Zeiser & Erber, 1977). It has been suggested that they do not *hear* at all, but instead detect amplified acoustic stimuli through vibrotactile receptors in their ears (Boothroyd & Cawkwell, 1970; Nober, 1967).

These two capacities for perception of amplified speech—1) auditory spectral discrimination, mainly on the basis of low-frequency cues, by the severely hearing impaired; and 2) (vibrotactile) intensity perception by the profoundly hearing impaired—differ greatly, especially when combined with lipreading for speech perception. Undoubtedly, an important reason for observed differences in the communicative progress of hearing-impaired children is the discrepancy in their *auditory* abilities.

Most moderately and severely hearing-impaired children are able to achieve high levels of oral communication skill because, under good optical and acoustic conditions, they can perceive not only place-of-articulation for consonants and lip shape cues for vowels through lipreading, but also complementary voicing, manner-of-articulation, and formant information through intact low-frequency hearing. As a result of obtaining through one sensory modality what is not available through the other, their speech comprehension by combined auditory-visual reception usually is quite high (Hopkins & Hudgins, 1953; Numbers & Hudgins, 1948; Thornton & Erber, 1979) and they quickly acquire oral language skills.

On the other hand, profoundly hearing-impaired children tend to experience more difficulty in speech communication. Although they also receive place-of-articulation and lip shape information through lipreading, amplification provides mainly supplementary cues to them in the form of speech intensity patterns. Voicing, nasality, and numerous postdental articulatory cues often are not apparent. Therefore, the important factor seems to be whether the child receives amplified acoustic information through his ears that mainly complements or, instead, only supplements* the cues that are available to him through lipreading.

The majority of hearing-impaired children live most of their waking hours in a multisensory environment, and, regardless of hearing loss, this probably is the best condition for overall language learning. Later chapters will focus on some ways in which children can be taught to develop their auditory-visual abilities.

perception and speech monitoring

Many hearing-impaired children learn to produce acoustically intelligible speech in spite of apparent limitations in their auditory self-monitoring systems. How do they accomplish this? Over the years, a variety of special instructional techniques and instruments have been developed to help these children recognize which of their speech patterns approximate normal articulation. Some optical techniques include: simply nodding, smiling, or gesturing when the child produces correct speech (Calvert & Silverman, 1975); providing cues for less visible articulatory features through a phonetic cue system (Schulte, 1978); allowing the child to watch a mirror for changes in his or her own oral/facial image (Pflaster, 1979); or providing the child with special electronic devices that detect and display a visible pattern analogous to particular aspects of his speech, especially voicing and nasality cues (Stevens, Nickerson, Boothroyd, & Rollins, 1976). Some acoustic techniques include: amplifying and presenting the speech signal through hearing aids to the child's ears (Pollack, 1970); or modifying the speech waveform in special ways prior to amplification, in order to match the acoustic signal more appropriately to the child's limited auditory system (for example, peak clipping, compression, vocoding, and frequency shifting) (Villchur, 1978). Some tactile

---

*Recent research suggests that much of the supplementary acoustic information contained in the speech intensity pattern is redundant with the visible articulatory feature of mouth opening (area of aperture) (Erber, 1979d). Nevertheless, this acoustic supplement can be useful to the lipreader (Erber, 1972b).

techniques include: allowing the child to place his or her hand(s) on the face or throat while speaking (Calvert & Silverman, 1975); or letting the child feel amplified speech patterns delivered by a single vibrator (Schulte, 1978) or a set of tactile stimulators, each activated by a particular sound quality (Sparks, Ardell, Bourgeois, Wiedmer, & Kuhl, 1979).

Our spoken language, although perhaps encoded and stored in articulatory terms, is transmitted acoustically. If a child produces the sounds of speech in a distorted or intermittent way, then even normally hearing listeners will not be able to reconstruct the child's intended message. Most of the compensatory methods listed above are intended to help the child judge the correctness of his own *sound* patterns, and so recognize and continue to produce speech that will be *acoustically* intelligible to people with normal hearing. To transfer this ability to everyday conversation, however, the child must eventually learn to substitute personal (or portable) feedback systems and self-judgment for the special external information (or instruction) previously relied on.

demonstration, perception, and imitation in learning

For a child to perceive and develop spoken language during daily communication, all available sensory information must be effectively used. Several authors have described communication methods that attempt to exploit a child's sensory potential (Calvert & Silverman, 1975; Ling, 1976). Both normally hearing and hearing-impaired children typically learn to produce speech through perception and imitation of a parent or teacher's speech models. Educators of the hearing impaired have followed this model by creating instructional strategies which formalize and/or systematize the demonstration-perception-imitation approach. They take into consideration the child's sensory capacities in the primary mode (normally, hearing), rely on audition when possible, but also devise ways in which secondary modes (vision, touch) can provide alternate avenues for speech learning.

For example, in one approach (Ling & Ling, 1978), you would examine the child's capabilities through the various sensory systems and provide speech models in a specified sequence: auditory, auditory-visual, visual (alone), and visual-tactile (see Chapter 9, Figure 9–2). When the child's *auditory* capacity is adequate for perception, *acoustic* models will be sufficient, and the child will learn to match his or her speech production to your utterances, even though your mouth is covered during speech practice (Beebe, 1953; Pollack, 1970). However, some speech features are difficult to teach successfully to certain hearing-impaired children through the auditory sense alone; in other words, their auditory capacity is *in*adequate for perception. In these instances, you would substitute optical or tactile cues such as those described earlier.

The following sequence is commonly employed in speech instruction: 1) the teacher demonstrates correct speech production; 2) the child perceives and attempts to remember this; 3) the child imitates the teacher's model; 4) the child perceives his or her own vocal output; and 5) the child compares his or her imitation with a recalled image of the teacher's model utterance and judges the similarity and thus the correctness of this imitation. Hence, development of speech through imitation requires the child to *perceive* the teacher's speech model as well as to *perceive* his or her own utterance.

Needless to say, you cannot observe the child's perceptual activity itself, and so you cannot teach this skill to the child simply by showing how to do it, that is, "how to perceive." Rather you usually would teach *perception* by the following sequence: 1) showing the child a repertoire of responses (or discovering those already known by the child); 2) associating a stimulus with each response; 3) presenting one of these stimuli with a request to respond; 4) having the child choose from among the alternatives; and 5) rewarding correct responses and pointing out (or ignoring) incorrect responses. If the child frequently responds correctly, you can assume that the desired perceptual learning has taken place. If incorrect responses are common, your conclusion is that the child is having difficulty learning, or that you have incorrectly presented the perceptual task. During instruction, you may vary stimulus and response complexity according to the child's success or difficulty with the perceptual activity (Erber, 1976, 1977a, 1980a).

Because the basic speech-perception process is not overt, but is hidden from the instructor's (and child's) view, most perceptual learning must be inferred. Even the child's degree of attention to the task often must be inferred from external behavior. In some instances, a child's head and body may be oriented properly, while in fact he or she is neither watching nor listening to the teacher. Considerable teaching experience is required to make correct inferences regarding a child's capacity for learning perception of speech, and thus production of speech, through each sensory mode.

It is obvious that speech perception and production are closely interrelated, although the direction of the dependence is far from clear. Perception and production are but two of the many components of learning spoken language. And so, subdividing and labeling teaching/learning activities into "auditory training," "lipreading practice," "articulation drill," and so forth, may be somewhat artificial and may restrict the child's acquisition and retention of not only speech-oriented skills but language itself. We need to develop methods that smoothly blend all of these instructional components.

summary

For both normal and hearing-impaired listeners, speech perception and speech production are closely related events. A child's ability to produce intelligible speech depends to a great extent on his or her ability to *perceive* its spectral and prosodic qualities. In order to perceive these qualities, hearing-impaired children must not only attend to the visible aspects of speech, but also attempt to acquire whatever acoustic information is available to them through their imperfect ears and hearing aids. They must learn, first, to perceive the correct acoustic speech model and, second, to recognize a correct acoustic imitation.

3

goals, concepts, methods

A principal objective of any aural habilitation program is to help hearing-impaired children learn to communicate through speech. Auditory perception plays a vital role in speech communication, during both reception and pro-duction. A child's awareness and acquisition of spoken language depends upon the ability to hear the messages of others as well as perceive his or her own attempts to imitate. A hearing loss in a young child restricts these processes and may delay or inhibit both his speech and language devel-opment.

main objectives

The term "auditory training" is used to describe numerous teaching methods specifically designed for improving a child's auditory speech-perception per-formance. Our intent is to help the hearing-impaired child apply his or her impaired auditory sense to the fullest capacity in language communication, regardless of the condition of the child's auditory system. Usually, progress is achieved through careful application of amplification devices and through special teaching techniques (Boothroyd, 1971; Goldstein, 1939; Lowell & Stoner, 1960; Pollack, 1970; Wedenberg, 1951, 1954). Our instructional procedures may include a sequence of systematically eliminating visible cues for speech, identifying auditory perceptual errors, and applying a repertoire of teaching strategies to overcome auditory communication difficulties when they occur. This chapter introduces both a rationale and a conceptual framework for applying many of the auditory evaluation and teaching techniques that have been developed.

It is common for language learning and everyday speech perception to take place through auditory and visual modalities simultaneously. Exceptions occur when the child listens over the telephone or attempts to communicate in an environment that limits optical or acoustic cues for speech. Although we are concerned here with an *auditory* evaluation and training approach to improvement of speech communication, other effective strategies do exist, and they may be appropriate at certain times for particular children. For example, in some cases a teacher may choose to encourage a child to combine auditory and visual cues for speech (Erber, 1975) or occasionally to emphasize visual perception through lipreading alone (Erber, 1974d, 1977a).

a general sequence

We will first consider a general sequence for auditory evaluation and training that can be applied to all hearing-impaired children (Figure 3–1). This simplified plan has been useful in guiding aural habilitation.

preliminary audiologic evaluation

A minimal audiological test battery should be administered routinely to each hearing-impaired child. This should include at least the following:

1. *Outer-ear examination.* The clinican uses an otoscope to look for cerumen which can block the ear canal or earmold, and also to check for obvious middle-ear problems (for example, perforated eardrum or otitis media). Cerumen should be removed by a qualified person such as a doctor or nurse. If the child exhibits obvious middle-ear disease, he or she should be referred to a physician.

2. *Tympanometry.* This procedure is used to demonstrate the effects of conductive hearing loss not measurable with conventional bone-conduction audiometry in severely or profoundly hearing-impaired children (Northern & Downs, 1978) (Figure 3–2). If a middle-ear abnormality is indicated, the child should be referred to a physician.

3. *Pure-tone audiometry.* When necessary, the audiologist should use an audiometer that has been modified by the addition of a 20dB-gain power amplifier to obtain air-conduction thresholds at higher intensities than can be produced by a conventional audiometer (Erber & Alencewicz, 1976). This allows the audiologist to specify audiograms of

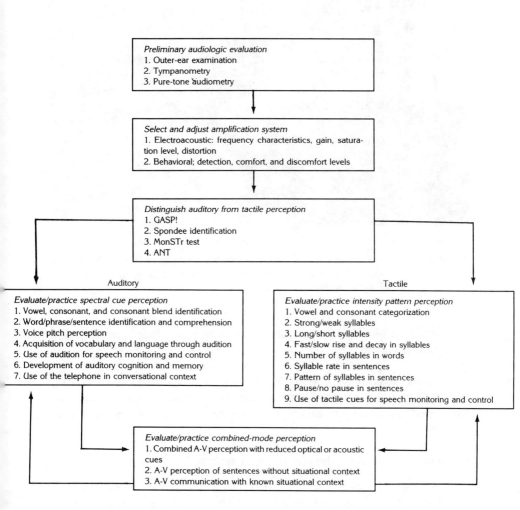

figure 3–1. A chart listing some clinical and educational procedures, organized to provide a framework for a general auditory evaluation and training program.

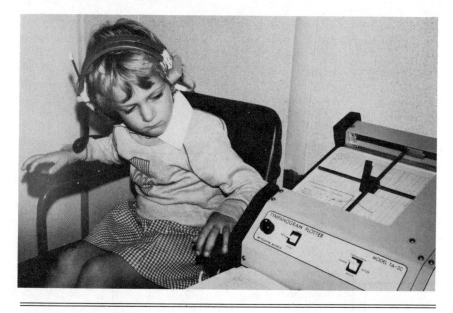

figure 3–2. Tympanometry is used to estimate the mobility of the eardrum as a function of changing air pressure in the ear canal. The resulting graphs provide information about the condition of the middle ear.

children with very poor hearing sensitivity, rather than simply record "no response."

These audiometric measures, although not incorporating speech as the sound stimulus, are nevertheless useful in detecting auditory factors that can impede (or contribute to) the child's development of speech-perception abilities.

selecting and adjusting the amplification system

An important step in any aural habilitation program is the selection and evaluation of an appropriate hearing aid (or aids) for the child. Without sufficient amplification of the sounds of speech, auditory training cannot be very useful. At normal conversational levels, some hearing-impaired children may not hear anything at all. Others who may be able to detect normal levels of speech, may be unable to understand what they detect. In either case, a hearing aid is necessary. One must remember that a hearing aid only makes the sounds of speech louder, not necessarily clearer, to the child. Nevertheless, without even this increase in the loudness of speech, a hearing-impaired child has no chance of interpreting acoustic information for communication purposes.

Hearing aid selection for young hearing-impaired children is difficult because they often have little vocabulary or language with which to describe their auditory sensations. They may not be able to tell the audiologist which of two hearing aids produces clearer speech or, for a specific hearing aid, whether one frequency response ("tone") or volume setting is better than another for speech perception. In spite of these obstacles, audiologists are able to select aids and adjust control settings for young children with reasonable confidence. It usually is not until the child is older, however, that the audiologist is able to verify that the early decisions were appropriate.

Several hearing aid selection procedures can be used with a moderate degree of confidence. 1) *Electroacoustic measurement* (Erber, 1973; Gengel, Pascoe, & Shore, 1971; Ross & Tomassetti, 1980). The hearing aid's output is measured electroacoustically and is compared with the child's detection and discomfort thresholds. Settings are chosen which boost speech to a comfortable level above threshold but not so much that the intensity is unpleasant (Figure 3–3). 2) *Comparison with previous cases* (Dale, 1962; Erber & Witt, 1977). Subjective judgments are made on the basis of clinical experience with other children who exhibited similar hearing losses. An aid is chosen which has proven beneficial to speech perception in other, com-

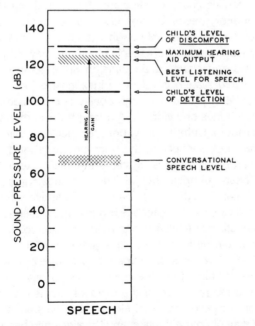

figure 3–3. The relation between various levels of speech that are important for hearing aid selection. Both psychoacoustic (e.g., child's level of discomfort) and electroacoustic measurements (e.g., maximum hearing aid output) are used to select an optimal hearing aid and settings for a hearing-impaired child (from Erber, 1979a).

parable children. 3) *Careful observation and measurement,* if possible, of the child's *communication behavior* (Northern & Downs, 1978). Both parents and clinicians observe the child at home and in the clinic as he or she uses a preselected hearing aid adjusted to certain settings. Basic test results, (such as speech awareness level), and subjective judgments are obtained regarding the child's responsiveness and speech understanding. Because none of these three procedures is exact, hearing aid evaluation should be considered an ongoing process, often continuing throughout much of the child's educational life.

Both the child and parents must be made aware of the importance of routine procedures to maintain a hearing aid. These include keeping the electrical amplification system in good working condition, replacing (or recharging) the batteries when necessary, and cleaning accumulated wax from the earmold (Craig, Sins,& Rossi, 1976).

What type of amplification system will optimize the child's hearing, speech, and aural language learning: wired, conventional personal aid, radio frequency, or infrared wireless; monaural or binaural; ear level or body worn? The benefits and limitations of each system are well-documented (Ross, 1977a,b). The *wearable* system is small, completely portable, and can be used both in school and at home, thereby providing "consistent amplification." Its electroacoustic characteristics are chosen and adjusted according to each child's auditory needs. But the child carries the microphone—over his or her ear or on the chest. Although the child's own speech may be consistently intense enough, the speech of others may be perceived with changing loudness and clarity, depending on distance and environmental conditions. The *wired* system is relatively inexpensive (per child), requires little maintenance, and provides a high-quality speech signal to the child either through earphones or a vibrator. A microphone normally is held close to the teacher's mouth. Unfortunately, both teacher and child are restricted somewhat by the wires connecting the microphone (s) and earphones (or vibrators) to the amplifier. *Wireless* systems represent attempts to optimize listening for the hearing-impaired child. The system is completely portable; the receiving unit can be adjusted to each child's auditory needs; a microphone is supported close to the teacher's mouth. But, present-day transmitter and receiver units still are relatively expensive, require costly maintenance, and may be cumbersome for very young children.

In general, *ear-level* aids are superior to *body-worn* systems in that clothing-rub noise is minimized, the microphone is relatively close to the child's mouth, and the presence of the child's head as a baffle can aid in sound localization. However, ear-level aids tend to be small and fragile, the controls may be difficult to manipulate, and the aids often become displaced from the ears of young children, especially during play.

Binaural amplification is considered superior to *monaural* amplification as it aids in sound localization, allows lower gain to be used to achieve a given degree of loudness, and allows each ear to contribute to the overall perception of speech (Ross, 1977a). Still, some hearing-impaired children have two ears with drastically different sensitivities and perceptual capabilities. Their binaural speech perception may be actually no better than monaural, and they may even dislike receiving amplified sound at the poorer ear.

Obviously, we cannot easily generalize about these numerous concerns of the educational audiologist. A detailed discussion of hearing aid selection is beyond the scope of this book (for such a discussion see Dale, 1962; Northern & Downs, 1978; Ross & Tomassetti, 1980). We must assume that present-day methods provide the best possible amplification for each child, given the state of the art. One can be sure that the content and quality of the acoustic speech stimulus entering and emitted from the hearing aid is extremely important, regardless of what sort of amplification system the child uses. To be effective, the hearing aid must be in good working condition, the room must be quiet, and the teacher's mouth must be close to the hearing aid microphone. Moreover, the teacher's spoken message must be timely, meaningful, and clearly articulated.

distinguishing spectral perception from intensity-pattern perception

A child's ability to perceive even simple speech material by listening alone at suprathreshold levels may not be very well correlated with the ability to detect pure tones during basic audiometry. In fact, there seems to be a considerable range of pure-tone thresholds within which prediction of speech perception performance can be grossly inaccurate. Therefore, actual speech perception testing is preferred as a method for assessing the child's auditory capacity.

For example, the difference between "severely" and "profoundly" hearing-impaired children is greater than just a 10 to 20 decibel shift in pure-tone threshold sensitivity (Erber, 1974c; Risberg, 1977). Most severely hearing-impaired children will indicate through their responses to speech that they can *hear*, although the auditory sensation may be seriously distorted relative to the norm (Boothyroyd, 1978; Pickett, Martin, Johnson, Smith, Daniel, Willis, & Otis, 1972; Risberg, 1977). In contrast, the responses of most profoundly hearing-impaired children strongly suggest that they perceive only the rhythmic intensity patterns of amplified sound delivered to their ears (Erber, 1974c, 1979d; Zeiser & Erber, 1977), and that the sensation is tactile rather than auditory (Boothroyd & Cawkwell, 1970; Nober, 1967).

It is crucial that the teacher establish early whether a hearing-impaired child can perceive sufficient spectral information, such as nasality and vowel formants, to identify speech components, or whether the child seems to perceive only intensity patterns (vibrotactually). This distinction is necessary in order to recommend educational placement, assign the child to an auditory-ability group, and plan the child's aural (re)habilitation. The audiogram may provide only limited information on which to base such decisions. Many commonly used speech perception tests for children, such as Word Intelligibility by Picture Identification (WIPI) (Ross & Lerman, 1970) or various phonetically balanced word lists (Numbers & Hudgins, 1948; Watson, 1957), can be inadequate for this diagnostic purpose also. That is, numerous children with demonstrated hearing capability perform poorly on speech perception tests that contain difficult stimulus items, such as monosyllabic words.

However, several spectral-pattern perception tests, can be useful in making decisions about aural instruction. For example, spondee-word identification tests (Cramer & Erber, 1974; Erber, 1974c; Sims, 1978), monosyllable-trochee-spondee identification (MonSTr) tests (Ballweber & Jackson, 1978; Erber & Alencewicz, 1976; Erber & Witt, 1977), and number-pattern identification tests (ANT) (Erber, 1980c) have been used effectively to separate hearing-impaired children into groups on the basis of their auditory speech-perception performance.

In each of these tests, the procedure is designed to elicit one type of response from children who can hear minimal *spectral* cues in the test words (although the auditory sensation may be distorted), and another type of response from children who can perceive only basic *intensity* patterns in the acoustic stimuli. Chapter 4 will elaborate on and demonstrate an example of this testing principle.

Vowel and consonant identification, as well as pitch perception measures, also have been suggested as tests of minimal hearing ability (Boothroyd, 1971, 1978; Risberg, 1977). Other auditory tests, incorporating both word and sentence material, have been developed to sample hearing performance over a wide ability range (Trammell & Owens, 1977).

auditory/vibrotactile evaluation and instruction

The preliminary diagnostic information obtained above allows the teacher to tentatively assign the child to an evaluative and instructional "track" (see Figure 3–1). If test performance indicates that the child is capable of perceiving at least some of the spectral qualities of speech, the teacher can direct auditory training toward identification of words, phrases, and sentences and also to improvement of auditory comprehension abilities (Grammatico, 1974; Pollack, 1970) (see Chapters 5,7,8, and 9). For example, the teacher might help the child learn to use sound for vocabulary acquisition, language development, articulatory monitoring, or auditory-only communication (as over the telephone).

However, test performance may suggest that the child can perceive only basic intensity patterns in speech and should tentatively be considered "profoundly hearing impaired." If so, acoustic (or vibratory) training directed primarily to perception of speech-intensity patterns should be provided (Erber, 1978, 1979d). The purpose is to help the child learn to recognize general characteristics of speech patterns, such as intensity, duration, and rate. Not only can acoustic pattern perception aid the child in lipreading, but it also can contribute to speech monitoring and control (see Chapters 5,7,8, and 9).

Sometimes a low diagnostic test score simply indicates that the child did not understand the test instructions, did not have sufficient previous auditory experience, was not paying attention, or was listening at an inappropriately low acoustic level during testing. Therefore, careful observation and repeated testing with speech material is required for a secure diagnosis. Thus, during instruction, the teacher should not present only pattern-perception tasks to a child suspected of vibrotactile sensitivity; a moderate proportion of time also should be devoted to listening activities requiring the child to make elementary spectral distinctions among, for example, voice pitches, vowels, and nasal/oral consonants (see Chapters 5 and 7).

evaluating and practicing combined auditory-visual perception

The final step in the general sequence is evaluation and practice of speech perception through combined auditory and visual modes (see Figure 3–1). This combined approach is the method that a typical hearing-impaired child will choose to apply during most everyday speech communication. Most likely, a child will prefer to lipread the speaker while listening carefully through his or her hearing aid. It is well known that, regardless of hearing loss, the child will understand speech better through combined auditory-visual perception than through either mode alone (Erber, 1975). For this reason, most teachers will emphasize combined perception whenever their intent is to present important new language structures, new vocabulary, or new concepts containing numerous details. When the purpose, however, is to provide special practice to improve perception through the auditory sense alone, then the mouth should be covered to obscure visible articulation, thereby directing the child's attention to the *sounds* of speech. Later, with the mouth uncovered, the teacher can return to more conventional auditory-visual communication.

Often auditory and auditory-visual practice can be alternated without serious disruption of the conversation. In other words, in practice, a skillful and experienced teacher can shift between the two modes quite easily, simply by covering the mouth during selected parts of an utterance. (The arrows between the final two levels of Figure 3–1 are shown extended in both directions to indicate this potential flexibility.)

a framework for auditory evaluation and training

The preceding section proposed a general plan to follow while providing aural (re)habilitation for hearing-impaired children (see Figure 3–1). Before discussing any of those procedures in very great detail, however, we must consider the various options that are available to us as auditory evaluators and instructors.

a stimulus-response model

Figure 3–4 summarizes the variety of *speech stimuli* (for example, words or sentences) that a hearing-impaired child might encounter in daily life or in a classroom or clinical situation. The diagram also lists the range of *response tasks* (detection, discrimination, identification, or comprehension) the child might be required to perform whenever these speech stimuli occur. We will use this matrix to guide our approach to auditory evaluation and training (Erber, 1976, 1980a; Erber & Hirsh, 1978).

Scanning from left to right in the figure, we see that the stimuli become longer and linguistically more complex. Progressing from top to bottom, we observe that the response tasks tend to increase in difficulty. A child's adequate performance at each task level can be considered a prerequisite for success at the next level of difficulty. For instance, a word first must be detected before it can be discriminated from another word. Also, several

SPEECH STIMULUS

	SPEECH ELEMENTS	SYLLABLES	WORDS	PHRASES	SENTENCES	CONNECTED DISCOURSE
DETECTION						
DISCRIMINATION				A		
IDENTIFICATION					B	
COMPREHENSION						

RESPONSE TASK

figure 3–4. The range of speech stimuli and auditory response tasks that occur during communication, for example: phrase discrimination (a) and sentence identification (b). This matrix is used to guide an approach to auditory evaluation and instruction.

words must be discriminated as different from one another before they can be identified and named reliably.

Each box in the diagram describes the interaction between a particular type of acoustic speech stimulus and a specific manner of response. For example, a child might be: a) requested to tell whether the two phrases *onto the books* and *under the bush* sound the same or different—a discrimination task; or b) expected to repeat (identify) the sentence *These shoes are too big for my feet.* (The boxes labeled *A* and *B* show the placement of these tasks in Figure 3–4.) Our observations suggest that nearly all daily speech perception tasks can be analyzed and placed in the matrix in this way. Both tests and listening activities can be easily created to fit into any stimulus-response cell defined by Figure 3–4.

Ideally, to completely evaluate a hearing-impaired child's auditory speech-perception skills, specific tests for each stimulus-response combination depicted in this figure should be administered. That is, before beginning auditory instruction, we should obtain complete descriptive and diagnostic information for every cell of the matrix. Noting which stimulus-response tasks seem easy for the child, we then would direct auditory training primarily to those tasks on which he or she demonstrates moderate or extreme difficulty.

But to obtain a complete diagnosis of a child's speech perception skills, a teacher or clinician would need to administer at least 24 separate tests (six types of stimuli and four kinds of response tasks) and several subclasses of each. Because this amount of measurement is clearly impractical, we tend to substitute subjective evaluation for careful testing in many cases—a valid and reliable approach when performed by experienced teachers or hearing clinicians. Some *specific testing* (screening) also can be very useful to quickly estimate the child's present level of auditory performance (Chapter 4).

stimulus materials

The variety of speech stimuli available for auditory evaluation and training ranges from very simple to very complex items. At one extreme are phonemes, syllables, and words, all of which are widely used in evaluative measures*. These brief stimuli are preferred by many people because: several can be presented within a short time; responses are easily scored right or wrong; the items can easily be presented within a closed-set format; and numerous speech-feature theories are available to help the examiner explain a child's perceptual confusions. The main drawback to such simple stimuli

---

*Phoneme perception tests:
(Boothroyd, 1968; Erber, 1972a; Pesonen, 1968)
Word perception tests:
(Cramer & Erber, 1974; Erber, 1974c; Erber, 1980c; Erber & Alencewicz, 1976; Erber & Witt, 1977; Hudgkins, 1954; Merklein, 1981; Quick, 1953; Ross, Kessler, Phillips, & Lerman, 1972; Watson, 1957).

is that they do not form the typical content of everyday speech communication, although a child's auditory performance with simple materials may be related to his perception of connected speech.

At the other extreme are phrases, sentences, and connected speech, all of which are very desirable as test materials because they represent the stimuli that a hearing-impaired child normally encounters in daily conversation*. The main difficulty with using speech materials of this sort is that the scoring of responses to large language units, such as sentences, has not been an easy task. Although many teachers and hearing clinicians feel that they should give a child credit for identifying the "main idea" of a message, it is much more reliable to score entire sentences or key words as "right" or "wrong." Also, a child may appear to comprehend an entire sentence correctly, but actually may be responding on the basis of only a perceived fragment. This happens because most spoken messages are internally redundant and somewhat predictable. Therefore, since any auditory response to connected speech material requires both perception of sound and knowledge of language, careful interpretation of test results is critical.

response tasks

Detection is the basic process of determining whether sound is present or absent. This response may take the form of orientation to the sound, establishing a setting for further acquisition of information from its source (for example, the speaker). Detection helps the young child understand that some things produce sound and that others do not. It is also important for indicating the relation between people or objects and the sounds that they produce. Awareness of ongoing sounds in the environment helps the child maintain contact with the surrounding acoustical world and alerts him or her to nearby activity.

Audiologists use detection responses not only in pure-tone audiometry, but also in establishing minimal hearing aid settings for speech perception. That is, a hearing aid must be chosen and adjusted to make speech at least audible to the child. In addition, teachers have applied detection tasks to determine which speech sounds are available to a hearing-impaired child under specific acoustic conditions. Some phonemes may be clearly detectable, others may reach the level of awareness only when strongly amplified, and still others may not be detectable even under the best conditions. For example, the teacher or audiologist may instruct the child, "Tell me if you can hear something. . . . / a /, / f /, / m /."

---

*Sentence perception tests: (Erber & McMahan, 1976; Fletcher, 1929; Kalikow, Stevens, & Elliott, 1977; Sims, 1975; Speaks, Parker, Harris, & Kuhl, 1972; Thornton & Erber, 1979; Trammell & Owens, 1977; Wilcox & Tobin, 1974).

Even if the child can detect a large variety of sounds, hearing is of little use unless he or she also can distinguish these sounds from one another. *Discrimination* allows the child to perceive the differences between speech sounds, that is, differences in acoustic qualities, intensities, durations, and so forth. With this ability the young child also discovers that different objects (such as bells and drums*) produce different sounds, or that the same source (such as a human being) may produce different sounds.

Same/different discrimination and generalization of sounds into categories are complementary abilities. To describe several sounds as the "same," a listener must place them into a common category. Moreover, the concepts of "same" and "different" can be relative, depending on the range of sounds presented. The words *duck* and *duck* spoken by two different people may be described as "different" stimuli in one context, but these words probably would be labeled "same" if they were presented in contrast to several samples of the word *apple.*

Often, teachers of hearing-impaired children use discrimination tasks remedially to check a child's auditory perception when he or she makes an error on an identification task. For example, presenting the original stimulus and the incorrect response together, a teacher, may ask a child, "Do these words sound the same or different: *seed . . . . fruit?*" The purpose is to find out whether the child cannot hear the difference between the confused words or merely does not know that the two sound-patterns (words) should be labeled differently.

Identification responses, commonly obtained in clinical evaluation, are simply labels (names) for what the child has heard. He or she indicates this by repeating, pointing to, or writing the word or sentence perceived. A teacher might ask a hearing-impaired child to "Show me the airplane!" or to repeat an entire sentence, "The children played football in the park." These types of identification response require the child to recall the stimulus in some way.

An identification response may be *specific* in that the child describes the stimulus exactly (—pointing to a picture of a dog upon hearing the acoustic stimulus, "dog"). Or the child's response may be *categorical* in that he or she identifies the general class of speech stimulus without specifically naming it (—indicating that one syllable is perceived upon hearing the acoustic stimulus, "dog"). Other categorical identification tasks include: naming the locations of acoustic stress in a word or sentence; labeling a sentence as "long" or "short"; or specifying the position of a brief pause in a sentence. These are examples of analytical auditory abilities that probably are generalizable to many language contexts and thus can be useful to the hearing-impaired child.

---

*"Ugh!"

Identification of speech stimuli is related to the child's developing awareness that objects have names and that these names can be represented acoustically. In addition, the child develops the concept that the sounds that objects or people produce have labels themselves (words) and that these are important for communication through speech.

Teachers use identification tasks to determine how speech is perceived by their hearing-impaired pupils. If a child fails to answer a question or follow an instruction correctly, you may ask for a restatement of the question or instruction. The nature of the child's response may indicate whether his or her problem lies in understanding its meaning or in identifying (or remembering) the stimulus sentence. In addition, special identification tests can be constructed to diagnose particular problems in audition. Test sentences differing in length, predictability, or syntactic form can be used to demonstrate how certain language structures affect a child's auditory identification performance (Kalikow, Stevens, & Elliott, 1977; Wilcox & Tobin, 1974).

The most complicated auditory ability, *comprehension* of speech, requires that the child understand the meaning of acoustic messages, usually by reference to his or her knowledge of language. It also implies that the child can acquire new information through hearing and can act appropriately on that basis. A comprehension response differs from an identification response; the listener cannot simply repeat what was said. Instead, he or she must indicate understanding with a response that differs in content from the stimulus, but is closely associated in some way. Specifically, if an adult asks a young child, "What is your name?" and the child repeats, "What is your name?", only identification of the acoustic stimulus has been demonstrated. On the other hand, if the response is "Daniel!", then the child has demonstrated comprehension of the question. Other examples of comprehension tasks include reacting to whole-sentence requests, such as "Give some popcorn to Liz!" or "Draw a picture of a house!" A word comprehension test may require the child to write the opposite of *hot, tall, happy,* and so forth.

Comprehension is a prerequisite for genuine auditory communication to occur, as over the telephone. Often teachers of hearing-impaired children informally evaluate their pupils' auditory comprehension abilities by giving instructions or asking questions with the mouth obscured (no cues for lipreading). Similarly, telephone communication skills also may be specifically taught as comprehension tasks.

common instructional strategies

Both research and classroom experience show that in order to maximize the acoustic intelligibility of oral messages, a teacher should use acoustically distinct speech elements, employ common multisyllabic words, and rely on short, simple, declarative sentences (Erber, 1974d). However, teachers must do more than present easily understood sentences to ensure concept learning; children's speech perception abilities must be increased by familiarizing them with complex language that they often may not immediately understand through listening alone. These two goals are incompatible to an extent, and thus teachers present instructional material in different ways.

Most teachers tend to apply one of two general approaches to acoustic communication. Some present ordinary sentences without much artificial control over the vocabulary or syntax; if the child does not understand, they repeat, emphasize, or simplify the material according to particular needs (Erber & Greer, 1973). This strategy typically involves the use of nearly "natural language" and the remediation of any observed difficulties. An alternative approach involves presenting vocabulary and syntax known to be within the communication capabilities of the hearing-impaired child; when the child demonstrates understanding, an equivalent but longer sentence or a question that contains more difficult vocabulary or complex language is supplied. This is an "expansion" strategy based on knowledge of the child's competence and on the introduction of increasingly complicated structures.

adaptive communication

A great many teachers have learned to combine both the remediation and expansion methods in the form of what may be called "adaptive communication". The stimulus-response matrix described earlier can be used as a model for *adaptive* auditory instruction. To employ such a model, you would consider each interchange of communication with a hearing-impaired child as a type of informal test at particular levels of stimulus and response. This aural "testing" continues throughout the day, with the child's responses suggesting whether he or she is functioning adequately at the level that you have chosen. With this procedure, each spoken message that you present during conversation will depend on the child's degree of auditory success with those preceding it. That is, your choice of communication task will vary according to whether or not recent stimulus-response combinations have resulted in the child's success.

If a child seems to be perceiving your speech with no difficulty at a particular level of vocabulary and syntactic complexity, then you either will maintain communication at that level temporarily, or you may *adapt*, by substituting new vocabulary or more difficult language structures. If, on the other hand, the child has great difficulty in perceiving a particular message, you may determine whether the problem is: the child's lack of attention; your own imprecise articulation; unfamiliar vocabulary or language in the message; the child's misinterpretation of the situational context; or a required response beyond the child's present capabilities. You then *adapt* by modifying the listening conditions in one of the following ways: by repeating; by clarifying or emphasizing some aspect of the original articulation; by substituting more familiar vocabulary or less complicated language; by redefining the situational context; by requiring lower level responses, such as *discrimination* or *identification* rather than *comprehension;* or by allowing visible articulatory cues (see Chapter 10, Table 10–1).

This approach is clarified by referring to the stimulus-response matrix of Figure 3–5. In general, the more difficult auditory tasks are located in the lower right corner; easier ones appear in the upper left part of the figure. A major auditory training objective is to help the hearing-impaired child maximize his or her use of hearing to perform the tasks in the lower right area of the matrix, those most related to everyday communication (for example, comprehension of sentences and connected speech). Initially, the teacher must test and observe to establish the child's present auditory capabilities and limitations. The boundary between "easy" and "difficult" listening tasks for a given child will lie somewhere between the upper left corner and the lower right. Most auditory training activities will take place along this boundary, with the teacher presenting a listening task at a particular level of complexity, observing the child's response, and then adaptively choosing the next task on the basis of the child's success or difficulty.

For example, during a word identification activity, you may name objects (*man, dog*), and the child must listen to each one and then point to a picture of each in turn. If the child shows no difficulty with this task, you may try increasing the stimulus length or complexity (*The man is walking, The old man is sitting in a chair, The brown dog likes to play with the boys when they come home from school*) while still requiring the child to identify appropriate pictures. Or, you may ask questions about each object (*What color is the dog? What is the man doing?*) and request comprehension responses from the child.

If, on the other hand, the child should fail to comprehend a spoken sentence, such as *Put your toys in the box!*, the stimulus may be simplified by presenting only the phrase *in the box*. Or, the response task simplified by requesting only identification: *Put your toys in the box! . . . What did I say?* In another instance, the child may respond *playground!* to the question *When do you go to recess?*, implying *when* was identified as *where*. In this case, you can simplify the response task from comprehension to discrimination by pairing the two confusing words and asking, *When, where: Do those two words sound the same?* These all are examples of adaptive teaching behavior occurring during auditory instruction.

Clearly, the effective use of an adaptive approach in auditory training requires: 1) an understanding of the elements of each communication task and the relative position of that task in an organizational framework (for example, Figure 3–4); 2) ongoing evaluation of the child's auditory speech-perception performance; 3) a repertoire of alternative auditory training tasks; and 4) the ability to consciously modify instructional behavior during communication.

SPEECH STIMULUS

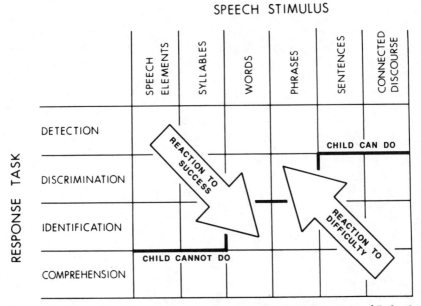

figure 3–5. A stimulus-response matrix illustrating the dynamic nature of "adaptive communication." The teacher chooses each auditory communication task on the basis of the child's degree of success with the ones preceding it.

summary

A general sequence for auditory evaluation and training encompasses: routine audiometric examination, including tympanometry and pure-tone thresholds; selection of an optimal hearing aid; auditory screening to distinguish children who can perceive spectral cues in speech from those who can perceive only intensity patterns; auditory and auditory-visual instruction according to each child's individual needs. An examination of each child's auditory abilities at several stimulus-response levels is suggested in order to diagnose his or her perceptual strengths and weaknesses. These findings establish directions for improving the child's level of auditory speech communication. Then, you can apply an adaptive technique in which you choose each spoken message on the basis of the child's recent responses and degree of auditory success.

screening
auditory abilities

Teachers commonly ask, "Where should I begin auditory training with Duncan, or Shelley, or Samantha? What should I do first?" According to the adaptive communication model described in the previous chapter, it makes little difference where you begin. Simply present several auditory communication tasks to the child (talking with your mouth covered), analyze the responses, and judge whether the levels of stimulus and response that you have chosen were too easy or too difficult. Then modify what you say (the stimulus) and what you expect the child to do (the response task). For an observant and knowledgeable teacher, these basic steps should be sufficient to initiate auditory training.

why test?

Most teachers, however, will prefer to evaluate the child's hearing abilities in a more formal manner before attempting actual auditory speech communication. In addition, most teachers will want to evaluate the hearing of each of their pupils in approximately the same way, comparing their auditory abilities to regroup them for communication activities.

Many special tests are available for describing a child's auditory speech-perception abilities and for pointing out the particular strengths and weaknesses exhibited. These include: phonetically balanced word lists such as the Phonetically Balanced-Familiar (PBF) (Hudgins, 1949) and Manchester Junior (M/J) (Watson, 1957); "rhyme" tests such as the Word Intelligibility by Picture Identification (WIPI) (Ross & Lerman, 1970); "easy" word tests such as the Spondee (Erber, 1974c) or Auditory Numbers Test (ANT) (Erber, 1980c); and multilevel tests such as the Pittsburgh (Craig, Craig, & Sehlin, 1975) and the Test of Auditory Comprehension (TAC) (Trammell & Owens, 1977).

Each of these tests is intended for a particular or general purpose. If the time is available, the teacher or audiologist may administer one or several of these to estimate a child's auditory capacity (Erber, 1977b). Each test has limitations, however: some are overly descriptive (and provide little diagnostic information); some take too long to administer relative to the amount of information obtained; some require special materials or equipment (test booklets, tape recorder, and test booth); some employ stimulus types, materials, and/or instructions that are difficult for certain children; some confound vocabulary and language evaluation with hearing evaluation; and some yield results that do not relate directly to a teacher's auditory training goals.

This chapter focuses on a method that you can use to rapidly obtain basic descriptive and diagnostic auditory information from each hearing-impaired child. It has been assembled in such a way that it fits directly into the auditory evaluation and training model proposed in the previous chapter. If you accept that model, then you probably will accept this simple testing concept.

The stimulus-response model of auditory perception (Chapter 3, Figure 3–4), suggests that there are at least six degrees of stimulus length and complexity, and at least four types of response task. As noted before, to completely evaluate a child's auditory abilities, it would be necessary to administer 24 auditory tests (plus numerous subtests to account for, among other things, variations in stimulus material). Clearly, this amount of testing is unreasonable; no one would have that much time available. So, instead, a condensed testing scheme is suggested to quickly estimate which auditory tasks the child can and cannot perform (see Chapter 3, Figure 3–5). Later, you will direct your initial auditory training to those tasks that seem to be just beyond the child's present auditory capabilities.

GASP!

We have arbitrarily* chosen to test at three specific stimulus-response locations: 1) phoneme detection; 2) word identification; and 3) sentence com-

---

*The choice of the three subtests is not completely arbitrary. Each type has been used before in auditory evaluation of hearing-impaired children, and so the procedures and typical responses should be somewhat familiar to many teachers.

SPEECH STIMULUS

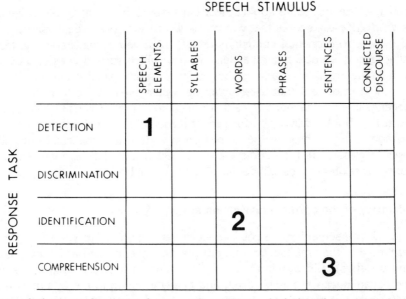

figure 4–1. An auditory stimulus-response matrix in which the relative positions of the three GASP! subtests are shown: Phoneme Detection (1); Word Identification (2); and Sentence (Question) Comprehension (3).

prehension (Figure 4–1). Three different stimulus types (phonemes, words, sentences) and three different response types (detection, identification, comprehension) are represented by this choice. This simple screening test is called the GASP!**—an acronym for the Glendonald Auditory Screening Procedure, developed at the Glendonald School for Deaf Children, Kew, Victoria, Australia.

The GASP! does not contain any unusual test items, nor does it require any unusual response behavior from the child. It does, however, require an elaborate administration procedure and is scored differently from most other speech perception tests. Performance is described not only on the basis of how many items the child perceives correctly, but also on the basis of the number and type of special adaptive strategies—the amount of effort—that the teacher must apply to help the child succeed. One might argue that this sort of test cannot be *reliable,* that is, yield repeatable results. Certainly, the GASP! is not appropriate for charting a child's annual communicative progress. Each year the teacher, and thus the examiner's voice, will be different, and the adaptive strategies that are applied also are sure to vary. Of course, a standard, tape-recorded version of the test would be more desirable for documenting a child's year-to-year progress, but then the adaptive com-

---

**The most recent revision has been dubbed, "Erber's Last GASP!".

ponent of the procedure would be lost. On the other hand, the GASP! certainly is *valid* since the scores that you obtain will reflect your speech clarity and also the environmental conditions under which you administered the test. After testing, an observant teacher will know which speech cues to provide to help the child develop his or her auditory communication abilities.

It is important that the *teacher* personally present the test materials, because it is the teacher's voice that the child normally listens to and learns from in school. Additionally, for similar reasons, this screening test should be administered through the amplification system that the child normally uses in class (wired, behind-the-ear, wireless; monaural, binaural, and so forth). Test procedures will be described in detail later in this chapter.

adequacy of the child's amplification system

Before screening the child's speech perception ability, you should determine that the amplification system (for example, his or her hearing aids and batteries) is in working order. This means, at the very least, checking the batteries with a battery tester, and briefly listening to the output of the aid(s) through a stethoscope for gross distortion, low output level, intermittent signal, and unwanted background noise. There is no point in administering these hearing tests if the child cannot receive amplified speech signals as intended by the audiologist who originally selected and adjusted the aid. If behavioral conditioning is attempted under inadequate acoustic conditions, the child will probably learn merely to guess randomly, and the responses certainly will not reflect his or her optimal performance. In brief, testing should not begin until the amplification system is judged to be working properly.

auditory detection of phonemes

The first section of the GASP! is intended to evaluate the child's ability to detect speech sounds. The test concept is patterned after the speech detection component of Verbo-Tonal audiometry (Guberina, 1964), and also represents an expansion of the Five-Sound Test (Ling & Ling, 1978). The detection subtest is given for several reasons: 1) to determine if the child's hearing aid is minimally adequate for auditory speech perception, providing enough gain and output level so that most phonemes can at least be detected; 2) to establish whether the teacher's voice level is sufficiently high for auditory communication; 3) to suggest whether the teacher can use acoustic modeling during instruction to correct the child's speech, because a teacher's acoustic speech model must at least be detectable to effectively guide the child (see Chapter 9); and 4) to establish whether it is reasonable to present the second subtest, Auditory Identification of Words. In the past, word identification tests have been inadvertently administered to children who demonstrated only much later that they could not even *detect* sound through

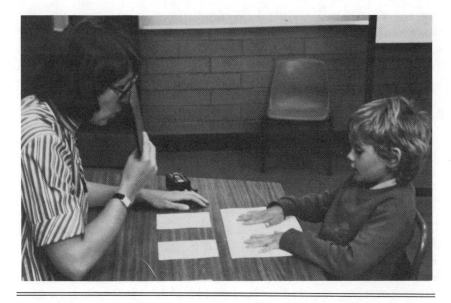

figure 4–2. A teacher uses the GASP! to evaluate a child's auditory abilities.

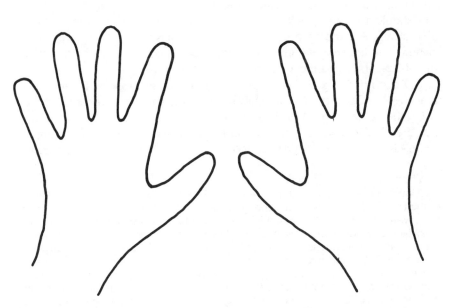

figure 4–3. Hand outlines that may be placed on the table before the child to specify a rest position during administration of Subtests 1 and 2.

the amplification system used during word identification testing. Obviously, the intent is to avoid testing speech perception abilities with inaudible sound.

standard test procedures

Placement. You, the teacher, sit opposite the child, with a table between (Figure 4–2). A diagram containing an outline drawing of two hands may be taped to the table top in front of the child (Figure 4–3). This indicates to young children where they should place their hands when not responding by pointing, and encourages focus on the task. This minimizes interpretation of ambiguous gestures. Usually you will not have to explain to the child the purpose for the hand diagram. Most young children will just naturally place their hands within the outlines.

Yes/No Responses. Next, place two pictures of cartoon faces with open mouths before the child (Figure 4–4). The two face outlines are similar, except that one face is drawn with lines radiating from the mouth to indicate sound production. The other is drawn with no such lines, to indicate silence. The picture containing the lines is labeled *YES*; the picture without the lines is labeled *NO*. In addition, the *YES* picture is brightly colored; the *NO* picture is dull black on white.*

List of stimulus items. You should construct a list of the vowels (no diph-thongs) and continuant consonants (no stops or affricates) as in Table 4–1. The list also should contain some blank spaces to remind you that sometimes you should form a speech sound with your mouth, but present nothing acoustically. A sample word is given with each vowel as a guide to pronunciation. The consonants are divided into groups by manner of articulation (nasal, lateral, voiced fricative, and unvoiced fricative).

Accompanying the list of speech sounds are two rows of boxes; these are labeled *YES* and *NO*. The child's responses should be recorded there, using the same mark (●) to indicate a *YES* or *NO* response.** Neither you nor the child should consider a *NO* response as incorrect; this response merely indicates that the child cannot detect a particular isolated phoneme.

---

*Previously, other pairs of pictures were tried. One pair contained two frontal views of the face, one with the mouth open (*YES*), and the other with the mouth closed (*NO*). With that set, the children quickly associated an open mouth with sound and a closed mouth with silence, as intended. However, if the child observed facial movement during testing, but heard *no sound,* he or she was likely to respond *YES* anyway, presuming that sound must have been produced. That was a serious problem, because one should like to present speech occasionally with normal articulation, but with no sound—to demonstrate to the child that this condition can occur, and that the child should feel confident responding *NO* when facial movements are visible but no sound is audible. Therefore, a pair of pictures that helps the child learn that visible facial/oral movements may, or may not, produce sound are now used.

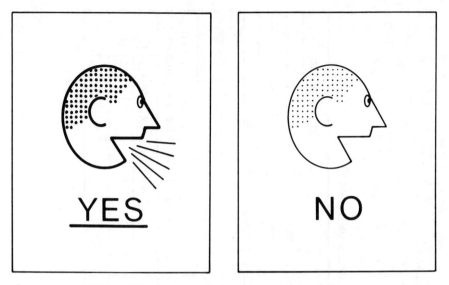

figure 4—4. *YES* and *NO* face-outline drawings used as response indicators during evaluation of a child's Phoneme Detection ability (GASP! Subtest 1).

Listening Conditions. Indicate the listening condition under which the test will be given by marking the matrix at the top right of Table 4—1 to specify the type of amplification system the child uses (for example, hearing aid, wireless FM, wired auditory trainer, or vibrator), and whether he or she listens monaurally or binaurally.

Preliminary instructions. Before administering the detection task, you must teach the child what is expected. That is, first say to the child: "I want you to listen (gesture to ear), and if you hear something (nod your head *yes*), point here (to the *YES* picture). If you hear nothing (gesture to ear, shrug shoulders, shake your head *no*), point here (to the *NO* picture)." These basic instructions can be understood by most four-year-old children after a few repetitions and examples.

Initial Trials. Next, ask the child if he or she is ready. Do *not* give any examples audiovisually; present *all* phonemes (or silence) with your mouth

---

**Previously, a circle was drawn around each detected phoneme and an *X* drawn through each nondetected speech sound. The children could see this, and concluded that this meant that sometimes they were "right" and sometimes "wrong." They usually tried to be "right" more often, by giving false-positive responses; they responded *YES* even if they did not hear anything. To minimize this problem, now the paper is marked the same way (●), whether they detect sound or not, thereby simply acknowledging their responses.

TABLE 4–1. A form on which to record a child's responses to GASP! Subtest 1 (Phoneme Detection).

GLENDONALD
AUDITORY
SCREENING
PROCEDURE
!

Child: _____
Teacher: _____
Tester: _____
Date: _____

How was child tested?   HA   FM   AT   V

	L	Bin	R

I. *PHONEME DETECTION*—Place dot(s) in the *yes/no* box(es) to indicate child's response(s).

	beet	bit	bet	bat	pot	bought	book	boot	but	bird	no sound	nas.	lat.	voiced fricative	unvoiced fricative
	i	ɪ	ɛ	æ	ɑ	ɔ	ʊ	u	ʌ	ɝ		m n	r ℓ	z ʒ v ð	s ʃ f θ
yes															
no															

covered. Gesture to your ear, say "listen," cover your mouth with a card*, produce the strong vowel / ɑ /, and then uncover your mouth immediately.** (Produce the / ɑ / with a loud voice near the child to ensure its detection.) If the child does not immediately point to the YES picture, move his or her hand to the YES picture. After the child points, repeat the / ɑ / sound, and wait for the appropriate pointing response. Next, cover your mouth and produce exaggerated but silent oral articulation of the vowel / ɑ /. Most children will immediately point to NO. However, if the child points to YES, say "listen again," cover your mouth, produce no sound, lower the card, and the child should point to NO. Finally, present the vowel / ɑ / or no sound for several more trials, requiring the child to point to the correct picture each time.

Verify task understanding. In these initial trials, be very careful not to *alternate* the / ɑ / sound and no sound. Also, present long sequences of each stimulus occasionally, even four in a row. The purpose is to make the child aware that even this might occur; he or she may be occasionally required to point to YES or NO repeatedly. You may even present an extremely long sequence as a game, so that the child can demonstrate confidence. Some children enjoy pointing to YES, YES, YES, YES, ... just to show that they are really paying attention.

After about a minute of this activity, most children will understand the task; they should listen when you cover your mouth and respond when you uncover it, regardless of whether or not you produce sound. If the child continues to misunderstand the instructions, you may try substituting a vibrator for the child's hearing aid, returning to the original device after the task is understood.

Test. Once you are certain that the child understands the task, introduce other vowels and consonants in random order, pronouncing the consonants as *continuants*, without an accompanying vowel (for example, say / v /, not "vee," or "vuh"). If you wish, you may present the vowels in the context of the key words, such as b*i*t or b*oo*k. Present each item at least once, preferably twice if you have time to confirm previous responses. You also should present "no sound" frequently, always marking whether or not the child detects each stimulus. If the child ever responds YES when you present no sound, you should supply reinstruction, contrasting a loud / ɑ / with silence. Continue testing only after the child responds reliably to this pair. If confusion persists, check the amplification system and/or the room for unwanted noise.

---

*The card used should be approximately 15 × 25 cm and should be a dull color such as gray so that there is little reflection of light. If nothing else is available to cover your mouth, rip the back cover off this book.
**The relative timing of card movement and speech production is extremely important. Don't place the card in front of your face until you are ready to speak.

TABLE 4–2. A form on which are recorded a child's responses to GASP! Subtest 1 (Phoneme Detection).

GLENDONALD
AUDITORY
SCREENING
PROCEDURE
!

Child: _____
Teacher: _____
Tester: _____
Date: _____

How
was
child
tested
?

HA
FM
AT
V

	L	Bin	R
		●	

I. PHONEME DETECTION—Place dot(s) in the yes/no box(es) to indicate child's response(s).

	beet	bit	bet	bat	pot	bought	book	boot	but	bird	no sound	nas.		lat.		voiced fricative				unvoiced fricative			
	i	ɪ	ɛ	æ	ɑ	ɔ	ʊ	u	ʌ	ɝ		m n ŋ		r l		z ʒ v ð				s ʃ f θ			
yes	○	●	●	●	●	●	●	○	●	●		● ● ●		● ●		○ ○ ○				○			
no	●							●			●●●●●●					● ● ●				● ● ● ●			

● = normal intensity; ○ = increased intensity

This phoneme detection task should take approximately 10 minutes. When you are finished testing, look at the pattern of responses (Table 4–2). Detection ability varies among hearing-impaired children: some children can detect all of the test phonemes through their hearing aids; some can detect all of these phonemes except the voiceless fricatives; others can detect most of the vowels, but only a few of the consonants; still others, only the strong central vowels / ɑ, ɔ/*; and some cannot detect anything at all through the amplification system that they use. (If this becomes obvious during initial instruction, do not continue testing, but instead try to solve the amplification problem.)

adaptive test procedures

After examining the response pattern that the child has established, go back and retest while applying special adaptive strategies. For instance, stress the vowels and consonants, or get close to the child, leaning forward to within about 20 cm of the hearing aid (or if you use a lavaliere microphone, raise it to your mouth) and repeat the vowels and consonants. The purpose is to determine if there are any special acoustic conditions under which the child *can* detect speech sounds previously not detected under reasonably normal acoustic conditions. You may try different tone or volume settings also and even discover improved performance with a different amplification system.

As mentioned, a few children will not be able to detect *any* speech sounds through their hearing aids. Although they may use powerful hearing aids, they may suffer from frequent colds or allergies (resulting in otitis media—inflammation of the middle ear, often associated with an effusion of fluid and resulting in conductive hearing loss) which shift their threshold sensitivity beyond the maximum output of the aids. Their auditory performance even may fluctuate from day to day for this reason. These children should be retested while they hold a vibrator connected to an amplifier. Try speaking into the microphone at various distances and angles to determine the effect on detection. (For example, the unvoiced fricatives can be made detectable if you direct you breath stream at just the correct angle to the microphone grille.) Typically, most hearing-impaired children will be able to detect nearly all speech sounds through a vibrator if you are careful to hold the microphone close to your mouth. In fact, many profoundly hearing-impaired children also can benefit considerably from *vibratory training—* practice in perceiving speech through a hand-held vibrator.

---

*Some children wear hearing aids that have peaked responses in the midfrequencies. The central vowels contain most of their energy in this range, and so all that the children may hear (or feel) is that mid-frequency information. Thus, they cannot detect / i / or / u /, which contain little mid-frequency energy.

Further, make note of *your* communicative behavior during the adaptive part of the detection subtest; this information will be useful during later auditory training. That is, remember what *you* had to do to help the child succeed, so if you administer a similar detection task to the child later, and he or she makes frequent errors, you will have recourse to past experience. The problem may be the child's lack of attention, the frequency response of the hearing aids, your voice level, the distance between you and the hearing aids, or noise in the room. If during previous testing, you discovered that shouting helped the child detect your speech, then you may conclude that the immediate detection problem can be overcome by that simple method. Obviously, a better solution is to decrease distance, reduce noise, or best of all, obtain a more adequate amplification system.

Occasionally, while administering the *detection* subtest, you may want to ask the child for an *identification* response—if the child is quick to respond, and you intuitively feel that he or she might be capable of identifying the speech sounds. Cover your mouth, produce the phoneme, and ask for repetition of what you said. In this way, you may obtain some additional auditory information very quickly. If so, you may think, "Why don't I evaluate vowel and consonant identification routinely as part of a more complete test battery?" Be careful! Next, you might even consider administering all 24 types of subtests and their variants! Stop and reconsider. You could spend all your time testing rather than directly providing communicative help to the child.

The detection information from this subtest will facilitate dividing children into very general categories. If a child can detect (at least) most of the vowels, it is reasonable to advance to the next subtest—Identification of Words. On the other hand, if he or she can detect little or nothing through the amplification system used, it makes no sense administering the next subtest until the amplification problem is solved.*

auditory identification of words

If the child was able to detect most of the vowels during the detection subtest, you may advance to Subtest 2, Identification of Words. The purpose of this test is to determine whether the child can identify words (in a limited set) on the basis of their spectral qualities, or can only categorize them by their intensity patterns. The results may be used to recommend educational placement or to plan aural development. The audiogram provides only limited information on which to base such a decision (Erber, 1974c), whereas the results of Subtest 2 often indicate whether the child can perceive spectral

---

*For example: 1) find out whether the child has a middle-ear (conductive) problem; if so, refer him or her to a physician; 2) obtain a more powerful hearing aid for the child; 3) try a tactile aid, such as a speech audiometer with a vibrator as output transducer.

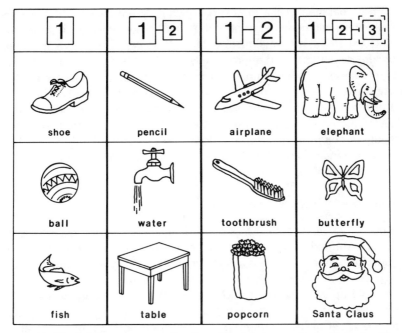

figure 4–5. Words/pictures representing four different stress-pattern categories. These are used to elicit a child's responses to GASP! Subtest 2 (Word Identification).

qualities in speech (*hear*) or can perceive only intensity patterns (*feel*) (see Chapter 3, Figure 3–1). Its format is based on the Children's Auditory Test (CAT) (Erber & Alencewicz, 1976), later expanded to form the Monosyllable, Trochee, Spondee Test (MTS, or MonSTr) (Erber & Witt, 1977).

We use a set of twelve word pictures (nouns) in this test, a convenient number for arrangement before the child (Figure 4–5)*. A particular child, however, may not be able to name all of the pictures in the set. If so, teach the words, or substitute other pictures**.

---

*This set of words has been prescreened for familiarity to 5- to 6-year-old American hearing-impaired children. A comparable list for Australian children contains the words: *hat, pig, truck; rabbit, water, bottle; toothbrush, football, ice cream; aeroplane, butterfly, kangaroo.*

**Be sure that the newly formed word set contains a variety of stressed vowels and initial consonants, and that syllables are joined by stop consonants, if possible (don't include both *doctor* and *bottle*; *butter* and *bottle*; or *lemon, orange*). Some three-syllable words will present difficulty in this regard. Very few have a distinct break between syllables, as in *but/ter/fly*. For example, in *kangaroo*, the last two syllables tend to blur, and in *elephant*, the first two syllables appear to blend. It may be necessary for you to say these precisely, carefully separating the syllables.

In preparation, place three word pictures from each of four different stress-pattern categories in front of the child*. These may be in the form of a printed sheet or individual picture cards. (You can make cards from parts of picture dictionaries and appropriately typed labels. Color-code the stress-pattern categories, for example, red for monosyllables, amber for trochees (strong-weak), green for spondees (strong-strong), blue for multisyllabic words, and brown for iambically stressed words (weak-strong), although these are relatively uncommon (*giraffe, July*).) Arrange the words in each stress-pattern category in columns, headed by a descriptive symbol (Figure 4–5). Clearly separate the individual columns of test words by dark lines, and shade each set with its color.

standard test procedures

Introduce stimulus words.   The hand outline should still be taped to the table as a reminder to the child. Introduce the test as follows: Point to a picture (for example, *hat*) and ask the child "What is this?" He or she should say "hat." Then you say "hat" while lightly tapping the picture of the *hat* once. Hold up a single finger and point to your ear to suggest one sound. Do the same for all the words in the column of monosyllables. Then gesture generally to all of the pictures in the column to indicate that they all are produced with the same pattern. If the child still does not seem to understand, tap his or her hand or ear while saying each word to indicate that they all are produced with one major beat.

Indicate stress patterns.   Follow the same general procedure for the other columns, indicating the appropriate stress pattern in each case. Eventually the child will understand that each column (set) of words is associated with the symbol shown above it. That is, all of the words in a column follow a particular beat pattern. Make it obvious to the child that there are four distinct word groups. Following all of these detailed steps, you should have little trouble administering this subtest. However, if you neglect a detail, or over-estimate the child's understanding during the instructions, the child may experience confusion during testing, and then you will have to repeat your explanation.

Verify word familiarity.   If the child cannot name a picture properly, either quickly teach the correct word label for the picture, or substitute a different word picture. The child should label all of the pictures properly before you begin testing. If a child's production contains gross distortions, such as *pop ə corn* for *popcorn*, try to correct the child's speech to ensure that he

---

*When testing older children, you may use more than three items per column (Erber & Witt, 1977).

or she has the appropriate concept of the word (for example, two rather than three syllables).*

Practice. After the child has named all of the words, give some general practice in responding. Make sure the child is paying attention, and then say one of the test words (audiovisually), for example, "Show me the.....*football?*" Then shrug your shoulders, gesture, and say "where?" (indicate that you want the child to point to a picture). If the child does not point immediately, his or her finger can be moved and pointed. Then gradually eliminate the carrier phrase, thereby clarifying the listening task. For instance, a profoundly deaf child may perceive "Show me...*pig*" as the pattern of a three-syllable word. Instead, wait until the child attends, say "pig" alone, gesture, and ask the child to point to a picture. Quickly, the child will learn to point to each of the familiar pictures very reliably, when you present its label audiovisually in isolation. The purposes are to familiarize the child with the general procedure and the location of all the pictures, and to familiarize yourself with the child's typical speed of response.

Test. Now you are ready to begin the actual test. Tell the child that you will say a word with your mouth covered. Then do so with a card, say one of the test words, lower the card, and wait for the child to point. Always begin this subtest with a word that is relatively easy for a hearing-impaired child to identify correctly, such as *butterfly***. The child's initial response may suggest whether he or she can hear spectral cues or can perceive only word patterns. If the child instantly points to the picture of *butterfly*, it is likely many other test words also will be identified. If the child slowly points to *Santa Claus* or *elephant*, he or she can at least identify stress patterns correctly. But if "butterfly" results in the child's pointing to a one- or two-syllable word, you may doubt that the child hears very well. After presenting the easiest word first (*butterfly*), you may present all of the other words in random order.

The child's response to each stimulus word is indicated by placing a mark in the appropriate square in the matrix shown in Table 4–3. Present each word twice, or perhaps even three times if responses to a given word vary—although always present each word the same total number of times. If the child identifies all the words correctly after only *one* presentation,

---

*The child still may be unable to correctly articulate *popcorn*, that is, imitate a correct model, after a brief practice period. When giving the test, you may occasionally pronounce *popcorn* as *pop(ə)corn* to see if the word can be identified more easily when you produce it the child's way. If you apply this adaptive procedure, make note of it.

**Highly intelligible words tend to be characterized by the following attributes: many syllables; syllables stressed; syllables joined by stop consonants; initial bilabial consonant, such as / b, p /; strong central vowels, such as, / a, ^, ɔ /. (Examples: *ball, bottle, popcorn, butterfly.*)

TABLE 4–3. A form on which to record a child's responses to GASP! Subtest 2 (Word Identification). A mark placed in box *A* denotes the response *fish* to the stimulus *shoe*—correct categorization by stress pattern. A mark placed in box *B* denotes the response *pencil* to the stimulus *popcorn*—incorrect. A mark placed in box *C* denotes the response *butterfly* to the stimulus *butterfly*—correct identification of the word.

II. WORD IDENTIFICATION

Stimulus

Present each word the same number of times.

Place dot(s) under each stimulus word to indicate child's response(s).

Response	shoe	ball	fish	pencil	water	table	airplane	toothbrush	popcorn	elephant	butterfly	Santa Claus
shoe												
ball												
fish	A											
pencil									B			
water												
table												
airplane												
toothbrush												
popcorn												
elephant												
butterfly											C	
Santa Claus												

Identification score: /

Categorization score: /

however, you need not say them again; obviously the child can identify the words under the test conditions.

Avoid visible cues. Never let your visible posture or head movement convey the word type while giving this subtest. To determine if the child is responding on the basis of visible cues, you may cover your mouth and present an artificial word like *pig-(ball)*, producing voice during only the *pig* syllable. If the child points to a two-syllable word, you may conclude that he or she is ignoring your sound pattern and instead responding to your eye movements or facial gestures. The challenge is to convince the child to *listen* rather than *look* at you for information. If the child consistently responds to your eye movements, stop moving your eyes, or try covering the *child's* face (including eyes) with the card each time you present a word.

Assign scores. After testing, assign scores to the child's responses as they appear in the matrix. The diagonal line indicates the intersection between

TABLE 4–4. A form on which are recorded a child's responses to GASP! Subtest 2 (Word Identification).

II. WORD IDENTIFICATION

Stimulus

Present each word the same number of times.

Place dot(s) under each stimulus word to indicate child's response(s).

Response \ Stimulus	shoe	ball	fish	pencil	water	table	airplane	toothbrush	popcorn	elephant	butterfly	Santa Claus
shoe	●	●	●									
ball		●										
fish	●		●									
pencil				●								
water				●	●							
table						●						
airplane							●		●			●
toothbrush								●				
popcorn					●				●		●	
elephant										●		●
butterfly										●	●	
Santa Claus												

Identification score: 14/24

Categorization score: 21/24

identical stimulus and response. Therefore, the number of dots appearing on the diagonal line shows the number of words identified correctly. The child's *identification* score is the number of dots on the diagonal line divided by the total number of word presentations.

The four heavily outlined boxes denote instances where stimulus and response have a common stress pattern. The number of dots appearing in these boxes indicates the number of words categorized correctly on the basis of stress pattern. The child's *categorization* score is the number of dots in the four boxes divided by the total number of word presentations (Table 4–4).

This word identification subtest takes about 15 minutes. When you are finished, examine the child's response pattern: some children can identify any word acoustically presented, without hesitation; some can identify only a few words reliably (typically, they will be able to name the three-syllable words and the spondees, but will have trouble perceiving the shorter words); others will be able to correctly categorize all of the words by stress pattern but will not be able to name them reliably; still others will be able to categorize accurately between mono-syllabic and tri-syllabic words, but confuse both two-syllable categories; and some children will just respond randomly and appear confused (unable to either count spoken syllables in words or distinguish strong/weak stress).

adaptive test procedures

After examining the child's response pattern (Table 4–4), retest using special vocal strategies. Find out how you must modify your speech to help the child succeed! Elongate vowels, exaggerate diphthongs, carefully articulate consonants, pause between syllables, or produce spondees with very equal stress. If any of these speech variations help the child improve performance, note the method used, especially if the child made numerous errors when you presented the words normally. Also indicate whether simple repetition of test words is an effective strategy. Two children may produce identical response patterns, but one child may respond confidently on the first presentation, while the other responds slowly even after three or four repetitions of the word. Thus, it is important to describe the conditions under which success occurred. Moreover, it is important to note if failure continues to occur even with extreme exaggeration; you may need to refer to this information later during auditory training.

Occasionally you will encounter a child who has great difficulty even in classifying the words by the number of syllables. In this case, try retesting, but first cover the two middle columns of pictures with a large card, leaving only the monosyllabic and trisyllabic words for the child to consider. Then explain to the child that he or she should listen again, but that it will be much easier this time because now there are only two types of words to attend to. Then briefly repeat the earlier instructions and retest the child. You may discover that the child can now easily classify the words and perhaps even identify some of them. Nevertheless, even under these conditions, a few children still will not be able to categorize the words and will continue to respond randomly. If so, either they do not understand the instructions or they simply cannot count acoustic bursts (syllables) reliably. They may never have been required to *count* detectable sounds before. This being the case, you will have to teach them how to do this—as part of auditory training.

auditory comprehension of sentences (questions)

Advancing to Subtest 3 (Sentence Comprehension) is recommended only if the child was able to identify more than about 50 percent of the words presented in the Word Identification subtest. Previous results suggest that children who do poorly on word identification are unlikely to be able to answer any questions at all and thus might lose confidence when confronted by this task (Figure 4–6).

Questions sample sentence comprehension ability in a relatively efficient way. Verbal instructions also could be used as test items, but in instruction tasks, the child may take much more time performing the task than is taken to present the instruction. Because questions are asked frequently at

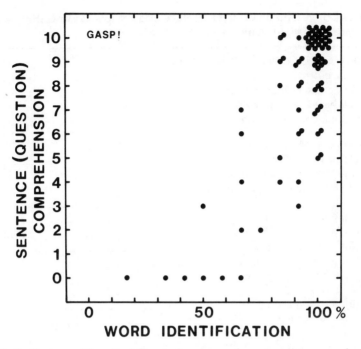

figure 4—6. Sentence (Question) Comprehension performance shown as a function of Word Identification score for 75 hearing-impaired children (age range 7 to 13 years). The GASP! subtests were administered as described in the text: each child listened through his or her own hearing aid(s) to the teacher's voice.

home, in the classroom, or over the telephone, questions represent an important aspect of speech communication. In fact, a question-answer format has been used to evaluate the adequacy of telephone systems (Fletcher, 1929), and several speech perception tests for children employ this type of stimulus (Butt & Chreist, 1968; Sanders, 1971).

Included is a list of ten simple questions, beginning with *why, what, where, when, how many,* and so on. The questions are limited to those that most 6-year-old hearing-impaired children can answer.*

---

*It has been established through trial and error that most young children can answer the questions listed in Table 4—5, provided that they know the content of each. A correct response requires only basic vocabulary, language ability, and general knowledge. Included are only familiar words and relatively simple language constructions, but not all of the questions are supposed to be *easy* to understand. If so, all children tested would obtain maximum scores and we could not differentiate among them. None of the questions can be answered with yes/no (We do not ask, "Are you a girl?"). No question is potentially embarrassing (We do not ask, "How much money do you have?"). All of the questions are relatively specific, to elicit only one correct answer (We do not ask, "What is your favorite color?"). Also all questions can be answered with only one or two words that themselves do not appear in the questions (We do not ask, "Which is bigger, a house or a bicycle?").

TABLE 4–5. A form on which to record a child's responses to GASP! Subtest 3 (Sentence (Question) Comprehension).

III. SENTENCE COMPREHENSION (QUESTIONS)			number of presentations	√ if correct (auditory alone)
Practice items (A-V): (a) How many fingers do you have? (b) Where is your mouth? (c) What color is the table?	Indicate: (A-V) _Emphasis_ _(Gesture)_			
Test items (Auditory alone):	Response	Comments		
(1) What's your name?				
(2) What color are your shoes?				
(3) How many people are in your family?				
(4) Where's your hearing aid?				
(5) When is your birthday?				
(6) What is your teacher's name?				
(7) What number comes after seven?				
(8) How many legs does an elephant have?				
(9) Where do you live?				
(10) How old are you?				
		Score:		

standard test procedures

The comprehension test is given without objects or pictorial prompts*. Place a large piece of cardboard over all materials on the table, so that a blank surface is presented. Then face the child and say, "I'm going to ask you some questions. Please tell me the answers."

Introduce task.   Present several sample questions (Table 4–5) audiovisually to familiarize the child with the task. For example, ask "How many fingers do you have?" audiovisually (without gestures). If the child fails to answer correctly, repeat the question audiovisually. If he or she still cannot answer, repeat again with some sort of oral exaggeration, such as stressing the words _How many_. If that fails also, repeat the question with oral exaggeration and gestures or eye cues to help the child respond correctly (for example, look at his or her fingers). However, if the child requires this much help to answer an ordinary question presented audiovisually, it is very unlikely that he or she

---

*The task can be simplified for younger children, however, by providing a pictorial context for each question (for example, a picture of a birthday cake for the question "How old are you?"). If you choose to do this, be sure to write down the special conditions under which you administered the test.

TABLE 4–6. A form on which are recorded a child's responses to GASP! Subtest 3 (Sentence (Question) Comprehension). The teacher's adaptive strategies are summarized.

III. SENTENCE COMPREHENSION (QUESTIONS)			number of presentations	✓ if correct (auditory alone)
Practice items (A-V): (a) How many fingers do you have? (b) Where is your mouth? (c) What color is the table?	Indicate: (A-V) *Emphasis* *(Gesture)*			
Test items (Auditory alone):	Response	Comments		
(1) What's your name?	*RICHARD*	*difficult*	4	
(2) What color are your <u>shoes</u>?	*blue*	*shoes→chair*	2	✓
(3) How many people are in your family?	*4*	*confident*	1	✓
(4) Where's your hearing aid?	*points to ear*		5	
(5) When is your birthday?	*Nov. 22*	*confident*	1	✓
(6) What is your <u>teacher's</u> name?	*Miss Powell*		2	✓
(7) What number comes <u>after</u> seven?	*4,8,9, etc.*	*"comes after?"*	9	
(8) How many legs does an elephant have?	*4*	*confident*	1	✓
(9) Where do you live?	*S. Kingsville*	*no problem*	1	✓
(10) How <u>old</u> are you?	*13*	*you→we*	6	
		Score:	*6/10*	

will be able to answer similar questions by listening alone when the actual testing begins. Regardless, write the answer on the response form (Table 4–6) and then go on to the next two sample questions. Finally, if, after presenting these samples audiovisually, the child still seems unsure, you may create more questions for practice and present the instructions again, being careful not to ask at this time any of the 10 questions that form the actual comprehension subtest.

Test. When it is clear that the child understands that you will ask questions and that he or she should answer, tell the child to *listen* to the questions and ask if he or she is ready. Cover your mouth with a card, including your nose so that the child cannot gain visible information from the upper part of your face. Then ask a test question as indicated, not necessarily in the order listed.* Lower the card, and ask for the answer. For instance, you may ask, "What is your teacher's name?" If the child answers correctly, write the response, give a tick (check) mark for a correct answer, indicate the number

---

*However, avoid sequencing questions that increase the predictability of the stimulus (for example, "What is your name? How old are you? Where do you live?") unless this is necessary.

of presentations before success, and then proceed to the next question (Table 4–6).

Remedial strategies. However, the child may not respond at all to the question. If this happens, tell the child you will repeat the question; then recover your mouth and do so. If the child answers, "Elizabeth," you know that the child has perceived that you are asking for a name. Adapt by applying a remedial strategy. You might choose to say the word *teacher's* a little louder. If the child still responds with the wrong name, you might try elongating the vowel / i / in *teacher's* or exaggerating its affricate / t ʃ /. After about five remedial attempts, you may decide that the child is not likely to understand a purely acoustic presentation. Try presenting the question again, this time uncovering your mouth only during the word that is difficult for the child (*teacher's*). In most cases, the child now will answer correctly ("Miss Fram"). If so, write the child's response, but do not give a tick (check) mark, because partial audiovisual presentation was required for success. Also, draw a circle around the word *teacher's* to indicate that you presented it audiovisually.

If it is necessary to emphasize certain words to aid the child's comprehension, underline them; if you present the sentence four times to obtain a correct answer, indicate that number along with any other important information. Thus, you should note whether the child was persistent and attentive during the entire presentation or seemed disinterested. Follow this same procedure with the remainder of the questions (see Table 4–6).

adaptive test procedures

In each case, you may choose whatever strategies are deemed most effective. A general rule is always to *repeat* first; you cannot be certain that the child was paying attention during the first presentaton. Next, you may try to emphasize particular words, move closer to the child, increase general vocal effort, elongate vowels, pause between words, or indicate syllable pattern by drawing imaginary lines in the air as you speak. In addition, you may present difficult words out of context. You might ask the child, "What did I say?", requesting merely a recognition response (the child may answer, "You said, 'What is your sister's name?' "). Or you can use synonyms, or present acoustic prompts. So, after the child says "Elizabeth," you might say, "No, that is your *sister's* name. What is your *teacher's* name?" Also, you might repeat what the child said and contrast it acoustically with the stimulus. For example, you may say, "*You* said *sister's*, *I* said *teacher's*," perhaps while gesturing appropriately. If you present all of this helpful information behind the piece of cardboard, and the child eventually answers correctly, he or she gets credit for the response because, although you applied numerous elaborate strategies, the child received no *visible* articulatory cues.

A child's answer can depend on perception of a single key word in the sentence, and its acoustic properties. For example, in "What is your teacher's name?", *teacher* is very difficult for many children to identify, because it contains very little low-frequency acoustic energy. Many children will perceive that you are asking about a name, without recognizing whose name is requested until you apply remedial strategies. Conversely, a child might be able to answer "When is your birthday?" correctly, yet identify only the word *birthday*. To find out which part was perceived, you may specifically request an identification response by asking, "What did I say?"

The answer to "What color are your shoes?" typically depends on correct perception of the word *shoes*. If the child misidentifies *shoes* as *seat*, *jeans*, or *boots*, you will need to clarify that word. "Where is your hearing aid?" also can be difficult, but for a different reason. The child may not perceive *hearing aid* as two words, with the first containing two syllables. Tapping out the syllable pattern for those words on the child's hand may help. "How old are you?" is commonly misperceived as "How are you?", if so, try emphasizing the key word *old*. Also, when you ask a child, "How many people are in your family?", the child may answer with the wrong number, forgetting to include himself or herself. It is important to determine the correct answer to that question before you ask it. Or, you may ask "Who?" and see if he or she names as many people as counted. And "How many legs does an elephant have?" tends to be a fairly difficult question for many hearing-impaired children to comprehend acoustically; *legs* and *elephant* may require clarification.

Nevertheless, many children can answer "What's your name?" without much difficulty. The question, "When is your birthday?" may result in answers such as "13," "August," or "long time." Likewise, a young hearing-impaired child may not know his or her address, so when you ask "Where do you live?", the answer may be "in a house" or "Bell Street." These are all acceptable answers.

With "What number comes after seven?", the child may say "six" because the word *after* is perceived as *before*. Try articulatory clarification. But beware: the child may have correctly identified what you said, but not knowing the meaning of *after* still answers "six." If you suspect this, you may gesture with your hand to indicate *before/after*. Or hold up one finger and ask "How many?" Then ask "What number comes after one?" (hold up two fingers), ". . . after two" (hold up three fingers), and so on. This acoustic strategy takes quite a bit of time, but it can be accomplished with interested, attentive, and persistent children. Eventually, the child may understand the meaning of the word *after*, answer the question correctly, and so receive credit for that item.

Above all, you should try as hard as possible to help the child succeed (answer each question correctly*) without allowing him or her to lipread.

---

*If for some reason, you choose to substitute alternate, easier questions ("What's your *dog's* name?", "How many legs does a *rabbit* have?") for those on the list, write the substitutions on the test form, and indicate the reasons for the changes.

Once you have given the child visible *articulatory* cues during the adaptive process, he or she cannot receive credit for answering the question correctly. Instead, your goal is to help the child obtain the highest possible question-answer score, using whatever *acoustic* strategies you can create and apply. You must decide whether your persistence is unduly taxing to the child, but usually, if you demonstrate by your relaxed manner that lack of immediate success does not upset you, the child will feel encouraged to keep trying.

In some cases, a particular child, regardless of how well he or she perceives speech, may develop an attitude of never responding to initial presentations of a question. Instead, the child will just sit patiently and wait, not putting much effort into listening, because he or she has learned that eventually you, the teacher, will provide additional (visible) cues. Thus, performance on the sentence comprehension subtest will reflect aspects of the child's general communicative behavior as well as auditory ability.

The child's score is the number of questions, out of 10, comprehended and answered correctly with only acoustic cues given. One of the benefits of this subtest is that, after experiencing its administration, you know, in general, what each child can and cannot comprehend at the sentence level, as well as the variety of special strategies that you need to apply to facilitate acoustic communication and learning.

With this subtest, it is possible for two children to obtain the same score, while one child is able to answer the questions easily without hesitation, and the other typically requires six repetitions and elaborate remedial acoustic strategies. One teaching objective for the first child may be to extend auditory comprehension abilities—for example, practice with more complicated language structures. For the second child, the goal for later instruction may not necessarily be to increase the child's auditory comprehension per se, but to reduce the need for such extensive, adaptive effort by the speaker.

application of the GASP!

The GASP! test results can help direct auditory training plans for each child, because the child's performance on a subtest may be very predictive of performance on other, related auditory tasks. For example, if the child cannot detect any speech sounds at all (Subtest 1), he or she will be unable to even categorize words into stress patterns. But if even half of the speech sounds can be detected (perhaps the vowels), the child may be able to categorize, and perhaps even identify words (Subtest 2) as well as some sentences. Similarly, if the child can reliably identify fewer than about half the test words (Subtest 2), it is unlikely that he or she will be able to identify or comprehend even simple sentences (Subtest 3). But if the child can identify nearly all of the test words (Subtest 2) correctly, this implies the capability to perceive the spectral qualities of speech and probably to comprehend at least some questions, as well as follow simple instructions acoustically. Finally, if the child can answer nearly all of the questions (Subtest 3) without hesitation, it is likely that he or she can perceive connected speech easily without need for many visible articulatory cues, and may even be able to converse over the telephone. In each case our general intent is to help the child improve beyond his or her present level of auditory performance.

summary

Despite the fact that there are many tests available to estimate a particular child's hearing ability, the results obtained often are not very helpful in determining the point at which to begin auditory training. The GASP! can be used to screen the child's speech perception ability at three levels: 1) phoneme detection, 2) word identification, and 3) sentence comprehension. The test quickly specifies which auditory tasks the child can perform when the teacher presents the test material and the child listens through the classroom amplification system. In addition, the test procedure requires the examiner to develop and apply a variety of effective remedial strategies. The resulting information then can be used to initiate auditory training with the child.

5

auditory
training procedures

three styles of auditory training

After you have used the GASP! (or another speech perception test, or your own careful observations) to estimate a child's capabilities and limitations, your findings will establish immediate goals for auditory training. For example, a child may be able to classify words (GASP! Subtest 2) into stress patterns only, but not identify any of them reliably. Although the responses suggest that he or she only *feels* the intensity patterns of speech, one cannot be certain from the test results alone. Therefore, in this case the child should be helped not only to expand his or her ability to perceive the intensity patterns of words, sentences, and connected speech, but also to attend to the spectral distinctions that may eventually allow him or her to identify these items.

Another child may obviously *hear* speech rather than *feel* its patterns, but can reliably identify only about half of the words in GASP! Subtest 2. Here the child would be given general practice in auditory word discrimination and identification, and these items would be presented both in isolation and in the context of useful sentences.

A third child may be able to identify words (GASP! Subtest 2) without difficulty, but comprehend sentences (GASP! Subtest 3) only after repetitions and the application of numerous remedial strategies. In such a case, one would help him or her to both identify and comprehend sentences (state-

TABLE 5–1. Three general auditory training methods.

Natural conversational approach:
   1) The teacher eliminates visible cues and speaks to the child in as natural a way as possible, while considering the general situational context and ongoing classroom activity. 2) The auditory speech-perception tasks may be chosen from any cell in the stimulus-response matrix, for example, sentence comprehension) (Figure 3–4). 3) The teacher adapts to the child's responses by presenting remedial auditory tasks in a systematic manner (modifies stimulus and/or response), derived from any cell in the matrix.

Moderately structured approach:
   1) The teacher applies a closed-set auditory identification task, but follows this activity with some basic speech development procedures and a related comprehension task. Thus, the method retains a degree of flexibility. 2) The teacher selects the nature and content of words and sentences on the basis of recent class activities. 3) A few neighboring cells in the stimulus-response matrix are involved (for example, word and sentence identification, and sentence comprehension).

Practice on specific tasks:
   1) The teacher preselects the set of acoustic speech stimuli and also the child's range of responses, prepares relevant materials, and plans the development of the task—all according to the child's specific needs for auditory practice. 2) Attention is directed to a particular listening skill, usually represented by a single cell in the stimulus-response matrix (for example, phrase discrimination).

---

ments, questions, and instructions), while gradually increasing their length and complexity.

As you work to help a child develop auditory capacity, you may choose from several general styles of auditory training. These differ mainly in specificity, rigidity, and direction (Table 5–1). Each style is appropriate for particular children and/or teachers. Each applies the principles of *adaptive* communication described in Chapter 3, but in a somewhat different way.

a natural, conversational approach

A hearing-impaired child usually will try to perceive the teacher's speech by watching the face and mouth while listening through his or her hearing aids. However, when speaking to the child during the day, you, the teacher, may occasionally obscure your mouth when turning your head to talk to others, or moving to write something on the chalkboard. During this brief absence of visible cues, the *sounds* of speech are still available. It would be of great benefit to the child if he or she could continue perceiving your speech even though the visible portion of your spoken message were blurred, fragmented, or simply not available.

As a matter of fact, it is not difficult to provide auditory training to many hearing-impaired children in just this sort of natural conversational setting. The purposes of such an activity are to give listening practice during connected discourse, and to increase the child's confidence in his or her auditory speech-perception abilities. To apply the method, you simply talk to the child as normally as possible, providing listening practice without specifically directing attention to the movements and positions of your mouth (Beebe, 1953; Pollack, 1970). It is not necessary to actually talk with a card or hand in front of your mouth, although you may choose to do so. Instead, you may stand behind the child as you talk, or sit beside him or her while working together. Specifically, if you know from prior experience that your intended message contains a word, phrase, or sentence that the child will be able to comprehend without visible cues, then simply obscure your mouth when you come to that segment and encourage the child to listen. After explaining why you intend to apply this acoustic technique, and after trying it several times, it should neither bother the child nor disrupt your communication very much. In fact, the two of you may even consider it an interesting challenge to communicate under these acoustic-only conditions.

Some hearing-impaired children have sufficient hearing capability to engage in conversation without lipreading for five to ten consecutive minutes with remarkably few errors. Others with similar hearing capacity can listen accurately for only a brief time, such as ten to fifteen seconds. But many other hearing-impaired children, whose hearing potential is comparable, perform very poorly on auditory tasks. They lack both the persistence to keep trying when they have difficulty and the confidence to make reasonable guesses. Instead, they tend to request, and depend on, auditory-visual clarification. Nevertheless, you will find that many moderately and severely hearing-impaired children can improve their auditory speech-perception abilities as a result of repeated practice in a low-pressure communication task. The skill even can be developed to an extent in a profoundly hearing-impaired child, if he or she has previously learned which words or phrases you might present in particular contexts. That is, the child can learn to identify message fragments just on the basis of the distinctive stress patterns of words you use in a certain context—"Jennifer blew out the candles on her ___ ___ ___."

Some children will obviously improve their listening behavior, and require fewer visible speech cues, once they realize that you are talking to them about a current learning activity. Every topic is associated with a certain vocabulary, and a child may reasonably expect only a limited number of questions and statements within that framework. Most children will discover how to use situational context to limit their choice of alternatives, and thus to increase their understanding of what is being said. For example, in the context of animals, an ambiguously heard sentence is more likely to be "What color is the mouse?" than "Carol is at our house."

Occasionally, you will need to find out what the child thinks he or she heard, by obtaining an identification response; the child may have heard only part of your message or, worse yet, may store an incorrect acoustic fragment in his or her auditory memory and later become confused (for example, using the word *thermature* for either *thermometer* or *temperature*). However, if you continuously request identification responses to confirm perception, you may break up teacher-child conversations and make them unnatural. So, you must compromise between developing a complete concept of language in the child and developing interest in listening. Remember that all normally hearing children perceive (and produce) language forms incompletely at first ("Dada work"). They eventually learn that the incomplete forms are wrong and that they must fill in the additional unstressed syllables ("Daddy is going to work"). Even normally hearing children will occasionally guess at what they hear during conversations, discovering later whether they were correct or not. If a hearing-impaired child answers a question incorrectly or follows an instruction inappropriately, then you can correct him or her, first acoustically, then audiovisually if necessary.

This natural, conversational approach is similar to that required in a telephone conversation; both require the child to receive information acoustically, without an opportunity to see the talker. Once a child has gained confidence in a set of basic auditory abilities, he or she may be able to use the telephone for communication as well (see Chapter 8).

applying the conversational approach

example # 1

Teachers can apply this procedure quite easily during most daily activities. For instance, an art teacher may place a child in front of an easel, and suggest that he or she paint a picture. Then the teacher sits near the child, so that he or she can hear while painting, and asks questions about the work or gives instruction. The teacher might indicate how to mix colors or might suggest how to complete the painting (Figure 5–1). The child may respond either by questioning what was said, or by simply following the suggestions if understood. Some children will be able to respond easily to acoustic messages of this sort; they may not need to simultaneously watch and listen to the teacher to understand the message. However, a child may seem to identify only a few words and may ask the teacher to repeat what was said after turning to lipread. In this case, the teacher may repeat while the child is looking and listening, but after he or she turns back to the task, the teacher can repeat or paraphrase what was said so the child can focus exclusively on the sound pattern of the message just observed. Or the teacher

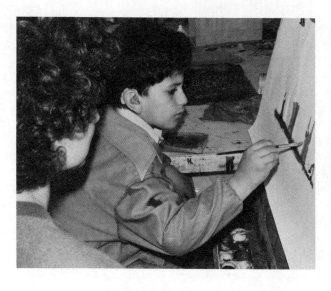

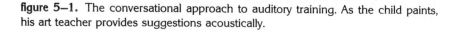

figure 5–1. The conversational approach to auditory training. As the child paints, his art teacher provides suggestions acoustically.

may present a different comment, with the goal of giving the child more practice in listening for the content of the message. This can be a relatively relaxed activity, during which a child's confidence in listening increases.

example #2

You, the teacher, can use a slightly more formal approach to provide a child with practice in comprehending spoken instructions. First, assemble or build a small object.* Keep it hidden from the child's view. Then describe what you have built acoustically, sentence-by-sentence. The child's task is to listen and construct an object that matches your detailed description. You should guide the child's performance as the contruction is gradually completed. Select vocabulary and sentence structures according to the child's responses and success with the task. The purpose is to help the child construct a car, house, farm, or whatever that approximates the original, with as few auditory-visual cues and gestures as possible. After completing the object, the child compares his or her work with your original creation (Figure 5–2).

---

*You can use the same general procedure with any creative activity, such as assembling a jigsaw puzzle, setting a table, potting a plant, making a notebook, or drawing a picture (Figure 5–3a,b).

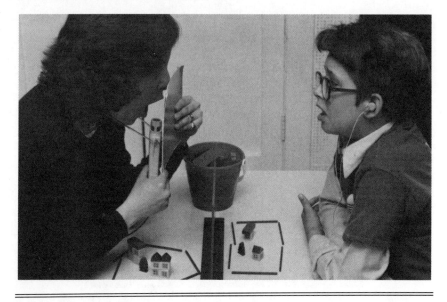

figure 5–2. A teacher describes what she has built to a hearing-impaired child. His task is to listen carefully and to construct a similar object according to her detailed instructions.

Many 6 and 7 year olds can sustain attention to this type of task for 20 to 30 minutes. The activity may be applied with very simple, individual objects, or with more elaborate ones. This object-construction task is well-suited to increasing young children's confidence in their own hearing ability. When you compare constructed objects after the task is completed, you tangibly demonstrate to the child that he or she can successfully comprehend your speech acoustically and follow your spoken instructions with accuracy.

example #3

A conversational auditory training approach also can be applied quite easily while children are occupied with desk work, as in a math class. The teacher can go from child to child and comment on each one's progress, or can ask questions about the work, without suggesting that the child look up. That is, you may stand behind or beside the child and try to provide instruction without visible cues, although perhaps occasionally pointing or gesturing toward the paper (Figure 5–4). It certainly will be easier for the child to understand your speech if you previously have explained, or pointed to, which item you are talking about ("the second multiplication problem"). If the child does not understand at first, try repeating or clarifying your speech. When the child finally is able to follow your instructions on the basis of

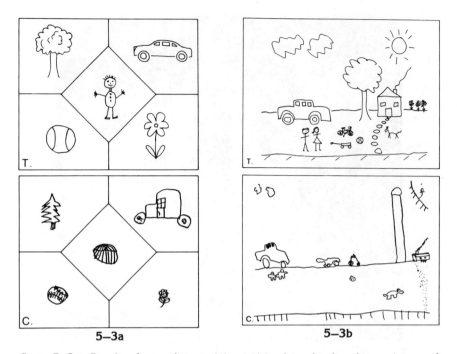

5—3a   5—3b

figure 5—3a. Results of an auditory training activity. A teacher has drawn pictures of five unrelated objects, then described them with mouth covered to a seven-year-old hearing-impaired child, who was requested to create a duplicate set of pictures (e.g., "Draw a ball in the bottom, left box."). The teacher's original drawings (T) are shown above, the child's (C) below. Note that the child has misperceived the word *man* and has drawn a *clam* instead (middle panel).

figure 5—3b. A teacher has drawn a picture containing numerous details, then described it with mouth covered to a six-year-old hearing-impaired child, who was requested to create a duplicate picture (e.g., "Draw a big tree next to the house."). The teacher's original drawing (T) is shown above, the child's (C) below. Note that the child has reproduced all of the objects, although some are not in the correct locations.

acoustic cues only, tell the child so and that you are pleased that he or she persisted. This not only informs the child that he or she did in fact hear what was said, but also increases confidence in *listening* to acquire information. Obviously, at first, a particular hearing-impaired child may not willingly follow a spoken request until absolutely certain about what was said. The child may ask for numerous acoustic repetitions for verification; patiently repeat and encourage the child to listen, especially if he or she seems interested in the task. Be supportive. Ask the child to take a chance and to venture a response. Explain that you will not be angry or disappointed if he or she fails to understand.

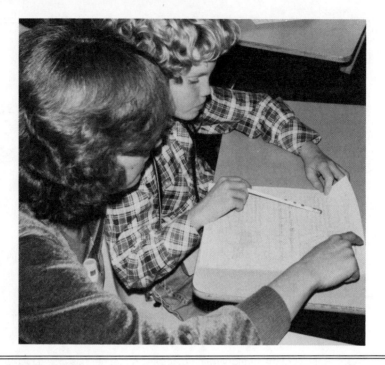

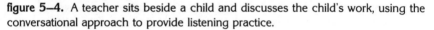

figure 5–4. A teacher sits beside a child and discusses the child's work, using the conversational approach to provide listening practice.

example #4

Opportunities for auditory training within conversation may occur while a parent and child are at the zoo. Rather than saying, "Look at me and watch what I say," and then, "I see a tall giraffe," the parent instead may stand behind or beside the child, and while both are facing the animal, talk casually and patiently about the giraffe. Other opportunities for casual acoustic communication without extensive visual cues might occur while both parent and child are watching television, cooking in the kitchen, or digging in the garden (Figure 5–5).

example #5

In many instances, you will want to combine auditory and audiovisual practice, using the natural, converstional approach. Thus, if you want a child to be able to tolerate increasingly longer gaps in the visible component of spoken messages, you can provide practice by systematically eliminating more visible cues as you speak. In addition, you might apply the technique with a child who lacks confidence in his or her auditory abilities (Table 5–2).

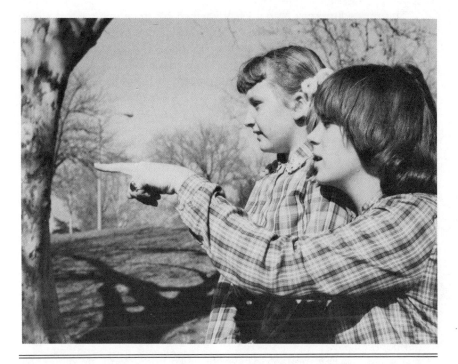

figure 5–5. A teacher kneels beside a child and talks about some ducks that they see on a lake. In this natural situation, she asks questions without providing visible cues for lipreading ("How many white ducks do you see?").

TABLE 5–2. You may help a child gain confidence in auditory perception by requiring him or her to *listen* to familiar phrases or sentences as you present them daily in the classroom.

Please erase the blackboard.
Put away your lunchbox (books, coat).
Where are the new batteries?
Did you feed the fish?
You did a good job!
Where is the red (blue, yellow) crayon?
It's time for recess.
It's time to work.
Do you have to go to the toilet?
What time is it?
It's time for morning snack.
Take out your reading (picture, science) book.

This procedure may be particularly applicable in certain subject areas. In teaching social studies, for instance, you may need to present information in the form of complete sentences, despite the fact that previous auditory screening indicates that your pupils hear very poorly and require practice in auditory *word* identification. You could present audiovisual cues for most parts of a statement or question, but eliminate visible cues by covering your mouth as you produce certain key words. Therefore, in response to a child's question, "Where is Ethiopia?", you might present most of your answer, "Ethiopia is a country in Africa," audiovisually but cover your mouth with a card as you produce the last word, thereby requiring the child to listen for this key item under acoustic-only conditions. Given the context of the sentence, the hearing-impaired child may be able to identify *Africa*, in spite of the fact that it contains several high-frequency consonants.

using adaptive strategies within the conversational approach

It may be useful to treat each of the tasks suggested by the stimulus-response matrix (Chapter 3, Figure 3–4) as component skills of comprehension ability. Thus, in the absence of comprehension by a child, you can apply a selected sequence of identification, discrimination, or detection tasks as part of your instructional strategy, and you can do this *remedially* as well as *developmentally*.

It is especially important to help the child understand the difference between the actual act of communicating and your detailed analysis and remediation of his or her communication errors. Rapid strategy shifts between stimulus-response levels are not likely to be successful unless you can confidently explain your intent to the child—"Don't try to answer the question now; just tell me what I said. What were the last three words? Do these two words sound the same.. . .? Can you hear this. . .?" Further, you will need to develop a special set of cues to inform the child that you are going to withdraw from the ongoing conversation for a moment and instead analyze your recent attempt at auditory communication in a special way. This sort of instructional behavior might be compared to that of a film director who interrupts a scene to instruct the actors regarding an interchange of dialogue.

It even is possible to incorporate adaptive auditory communication into interactive classroom conversation if the group is fairly homogeneous with regard to hearing capacity, and if the teacher does not devote an excessive amount of time to remedial strategies. For example, in the course of a discussion, you may cover your mouth and explain to a child, "The girl said, 'Good afternoon!'." If the child indicates a lack of comprehension, you may shift to an identification task and instruct, "Say what I say: The girl said, 'Good afternoon!'." If the child responds, "The boy ate a big extra meal," then you might quickly try a simple discrimination activity, comparing the words *boy* and *girl* and/or the phrases *big extra meal* and *good afternoon*. The child must listen and determine whether these pairs sound the same or different

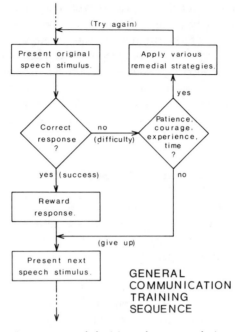

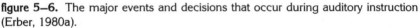

figure 5–6. The major events and decisions that occur during auditory instruction (Erber, 1980a).

before you reevaluate his or her comprehension of the original statement. The entire remedial sequence may be accomplished in about thirty seconds, provided that the child is familiar with the procedural sequence routinely used at each level.

Figure 5–6 summarizes the sequence, exemplified above, that many teachers typically follow while incorporating auditory speech-perception tasks into conversation. You would begin the process by covering your mouth to eliminate visible cues and then presenting an instruction or question to the child. If the child responds correctly to this informal auditory test, you, the teacher, will reward the child's successful speech comprehension and will continue the acoustic conversation. If the child consistently comprehends your speech with no difficulty at the particular level of vocabulary and/or syntactic complexity that you have chosen, you either will maintain acoustic communication at that level, or you will consciously adapt to the child's (and your) success by substituting new vocabulary or more difficult language structures.

If, on the contrary, the child demonstrates difficulty in comprehending your acoustic message and either responds incorrectly or fails to respond, analyze the situation and decide whether to bypass the auditory error ("give up") and simply proceed with the conversation, or to attempt remedial instruction. Your decision will depend on your auditory training experience as well as on the amount of time available. You may *adapt* to the auditory communication difficulty in several ways, by: repeating all or part of the utterance; clarifying or emphasizing some aspect of articulation; decreasing the complexity of vocabulary or language in the message; redefining the situational context; or allowing visual perception of part or all of the utterance (Erber & Greer, 1973). You may follow this remediation cycle several times, as you modify the stimulus complexity and/or the response task during practice activities and finally return to retest, or reexamine the child's comprehension of your original utterance.

a moderately structured approach

Even if a child has considerable hearing, the teacher must consciously use adaptive procedures to insure the success of a natural, conversational approach. That is, the teacher must keep the stimulus-response model in mind while communicating with the child, and adapt to the child's present responses by varying the difficulty of future auditory tasks. Adherence to the conversational method requires a clear theoretical understanding of the adaptive communication model, an awareness of the child's speech perception abilities, and control over one's own communicative behavior. Because initially some inexperienced teachers cannot manage all of these factors at once, and need a more directed approach to auditory training, a Simplified Classroom Sequence (Figure 5–7) has been established. Nearly anyone, regardless of teaching experience, can apply auditory training successfully by following this moderately structured plan.

This type of auditory training is a bit more formal than the natural conversational approach just described, but it still can be organized as an open-ended activity. The method is based on the "experience chart-story" format developed by Simmons (1968, 1971), after Groht's (1958) early work, which later was extended by Golf (1970), Moog (1970), and others. The original intent of the procedure was not to provide listening practice per se but to help a child associate spoken language with recent home or class experiences.

a simplified classroom sequence

Now let us look at the sequence of steps illustrated in Figure 5–7. First, you, the teacher, should participate with the children in some sort of activity (Figure 5–8a,b,c,). This can take the form of a preplanned formal excursion, such as a tour through a nearby factory, or the activity can be so casual and unanticipated that you may even think it is inappropriate as a source of material for auditory training, for example, going outside for recess, climbing a tree, and returning. After the shared experience, you should talk about it with the children. Depending on how much time is available, *you* may choose

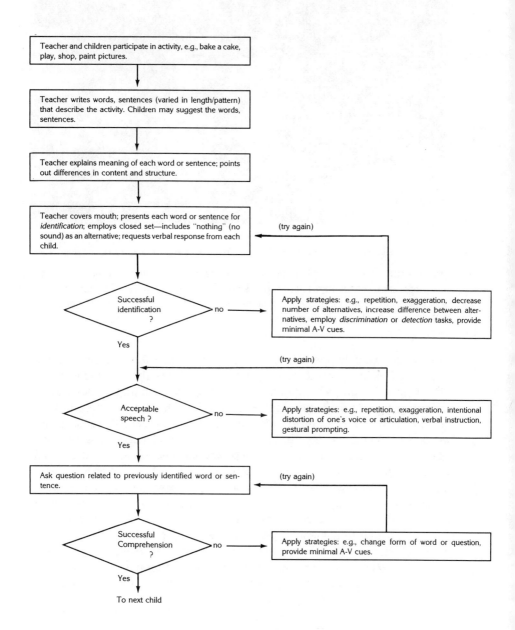

figure 5–7. A simplified classroom sequence for auditory training.

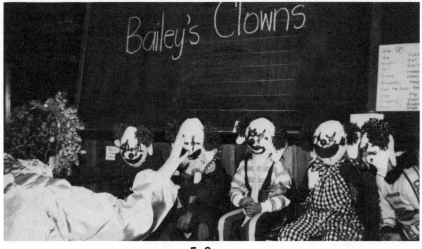

5–8a.

figure 5–8a. A teacher and her class of young hearing-impaired children participate in a preplanned activity, an afternoon "clown party," at which the children dress as clowns, do circus tricks, and eat ice cream and candy. Here, the teacher describes to the class what they will do next.

to describe what happened, or you can ask the *children* to provide the narration. Based on this discussion, write a set of descriptive sentences that differ in length, complexity, pitch variation, intensity pattern, vocabulary, and so forth in order to make these sentences moderately easy to identify through audition alone. The degree to which the sentences should differ acoustically will depend on the hearing abilities of the children and their prior experience with listening tasks of this sort.* Even profoundly hearing-impaired children can easily participate in this type of perceptual activity if the sentence patterns are made sufficiently different. You should experiment with different degrees of sentence similarity to determine how variations in pattern and content affect the children's interest, motivation, and ultimate auditory success.

In addition to sentences, you might want to include important words in the set, such as the names of children or objects that played an important role in the activity. All words and sentences should be numbered, and one of the alternatives should be blank (the teacher covers the mouth, articulates,

---

*Don't worry if you do not produce distinguishable sentences on your first few attempts. With the adaptive procedure, you can consider the task as a "test" for the children, and later modify the sentences on the basis of their responses.

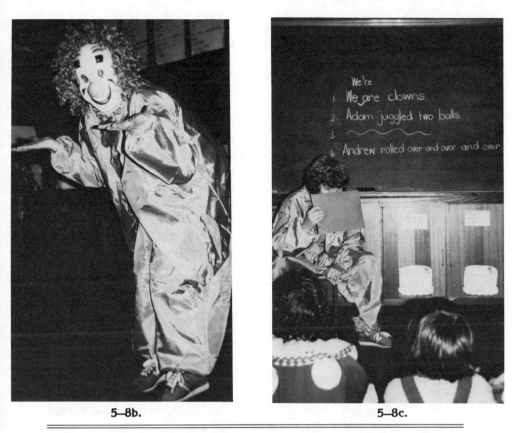

5—8b.

5—8c.

figure 5—8b. The teacher reviews the afternoon's activities while still in costume. In this unique way, she presents information without visible cues for speech.

figure 5—8c. The teacher has written a brief set of sentences that describe some things that happened during the "clown party." She presents each one (without visible articulatory cues) for identification by the children.

but produces no sound)*. In some instances, you may want to construct sentences with moderate attention to length or pattern, as shown in Table

---

*The purpose for including *nothing* as a response alternative is to allow the child the opportunity to tell you that he or she cannot hear anything (for example, the hearing aid may be defective). If the child indicates that he or she hears *nothing* when you have produced one of the voiced stimuli (word or sentence), you may wish to apply an adaptive strategy (for example, check the hearing aid battery, repeat, speak louder). If you discover that the battery is weak, don't be angry with the child for not replacing it earlier; be happy that he or she has informed you by responding correctly. Occasionally, also, you may present nothing to assure yourself that the child remembers how to react in such a case.

5–3. In this case, only a small amount of effort is required to list sentences that differ in number of syllables, number and location of pauses (as between phrases and clauses), and content.

In other instances, you may want to construct sentences more carefully for special purposes. This takes more time and effort. Table 5–4 presents a set of sentences that were used to exemplify length differences (at least in terms of length of the printed message). This response form, placed in front of the child, clearly shows the gradations in length within the response set.

At still other times, you may choose to group sentences by pattern and structure, as shown in Table 5–5. With this approach, profoundly hearing-impaired children are able to practice categorizing sentence patterns, while moderately and severely hearing-impaired children, who hear well enough to recognize constituent words, can practice identifying specific sentences.

Before beginning listening practice, it can be very helpful to point out differences in the structure and content of the sentences to the children, especially for those (profoundly hearing-impaired) children who depend on pattern perception. There are various ways to do this. As far as *structure* is concerned, you can use colored chalk to mark the periods that denote long pauses at the ends of sentences, the commas that indicate brief pauses, and also the blank sentence (no sound). Lines can be drawn under major units to emphasize the intensity patterns: for example a long line indicates a long sentence, two short lines denote a two-syllable word. You may add accent marks also, but some younger children do not yet know what they mean; however, nearly all children quickly learn that line length is analogous to duration. When you read the sentences to the class, "act out" the special markings—cover your mouth and move your hand under the sentence while saying the words, when you come to a pause or a period, hold up your hand to indicate "stop talking here."

Furthermore, it is important to describe the *content* of the sentences, the specific words, even for those children who have minimal hearing capacity. A picture showing the event or object may be drawn beside each word or sentence for this purpose. You may point out key words both for children who can and cannot read; some children may be able to read key words fluently, but not the entire sentence. In any event, it is best to briefly describe both *content* and *structure* of all sentences, since many classes contain children with a range of hearing abilities.

Expanding upon the content/structure description, you may explain why you think these written items are important choices, considering the shared class experiences they describe. You may even elaborate and present this as a language-development activity. How much time you devote to this step is your decision.

Some teachers can exploit any common unplanned event that occurs, even a routine walk down the hall, creating an auditory training activity from

TABLE 5–3. A set of words and sentences from an experience story intended for auditory training. This set contains sound stimuli whose patterns are quite different from one another. Even if the hearing-impaired children can only detect vowels, they should be able to distinguish these items without difficulty.

> *WE WENT OUTSIDE*
> 1. It rained, but we went outside for recess anyway. (a long sentence)
> 2. Nick got wet. (a short sentence)
> 3. Five birds sat in a tree. They were singing. (two short sentences)
> 4. (*nothing*)
> 5. playground (a spondaic word)
> 6. boots (a monosyllabic word)

TABLE 5–4. A set of sentences constructed for use in an auditory identification task. These sentences are formed and listed in this way to indicate pattern and length differences.

> 1. Mark laughed.
> 2. Yvonne likes horses.
> 3. Maria wrote a long letter.
> 4. Today, two men will fix the roof.
> 5. Glenn keeps all of his stamps in a book.
> 6. Barry cut up some vegetables. Then he made a salad.
> 7. Every morning at 7:00 o'clock, the children eat breakfast together.

TABLE 5–5. A set of sentences grouped according to intensity pattern: a) unbroken pattern; b) initial stressed word, followed by a brief pause; c) introductory phrase, followed by a brief pause. Children may practice either auditory identification of specific sentences, or categorization of the sentences into general pattern classes.

> **a.** (_____)
> My teacher bought apples at the shop.
> The children played football in the park.
> We put our papers on the bookshelf.
> We saw three elephants at the zoo.
> **b.** (_____) (_____)
> Rrrrr! We heard a fire truck on High Street.
> Crash! Trudy dropped all the dirty plates.
> Hey! You forgot to tie your shoes.
> Ouch! I bumped my head on the car door.
> **c.** (_____) (_____)
> After playtime, we drank some cold juice.
> For breakfast, we ate bacon and eggs.
> In the box, there are twelve new pencils.
> Under the tree, we found a lizard.

a description of that experience.* This is possible once the children gain familiarity with listening activities in general, learn the specific instructional procedures that the teacher will apply, and can anticipate what is expected of them. That is, when they see you write a set of sentences on the chalkboard, they know it is time to talk about a recent experience and then *listen* to you briefly describe the events.

Once you have written and discussed the sentences that you will present for practice, inform the class that they are going to listen to these sentences. You may do this most efficiently by selecting one child to be a listener, telling the others to listen also and to judge whether or not the chosen child is correct. When this child comes before the class, cover your mouth and say one of the speech samples; the child then repeats the sentence as accurately as possible. Ask the class if the child was correct. If he or she made an identification error, you must apply remedial strategies—say the sentence again, ask the child to listen more carefully, or exaggerate the sentence. In some cases, it may be necessary to decrease the number of response alternatives; you might tell the child to choose from only the top three sentences, covering the bottom three alternatives as a reminder. Also, if necessary, you might provide a visible articulatory (lipreading) cue. (If the child responds correctly, he or she has not succeeded at an *auditory* task; but at least the proper type of response has been learned.) In summary, you should quickly try several strategies until the child can identify the word or sentence and repeat it (Figure 5–7).

Next, you should decide whether the child's speech was acceptable when repeating the word or sentence. That decision is somewhat arbitrary, as your criteria will change from child to child, and from day to day. The child's speech quality also will depend on the sentences; some will be long while others may contain difficult words. Another factor is the amount of time for this particular learning activity. If you judge that the child's speech is unacceptable, try a variety of the strategies described in Chapter 9.

After the child has made several attempts at speech improvement, find out whether or not he or she can answer a question relating to the sentence. For example, if you presented the word *boots* and the child identified it correctly, you might then ask, "What color are your boots?" If the child can answer the question, then let another child have a turn as chosen listener. But, if the child *cannot* answer the question, you should employ various strategies—changing the form of the question, or providing a visible cue— until the child answers correctly. Then give the next child a turn.

---

*1. We walked to the art room.
2. Stephanie ran.
3. We saw the children in Mrs. Oakley's room. They were reading.
4. (nothing)

If you follow this procedure, you can convert this moderately con-strained activity into a kind of simple conversation. While the time spent with each child will vary, they all will receive your personal attention for a few minutes. Although some children, especially younger ones, may take several weeks to learn the sequence, after about a week of practice, *you* probably will feel very confident in applying and adapting the procedure.

For the teacher, the hardest thing to learn is how to construct sentences and/or choose words which will sound different to hearing-impaired children. Although your written sentences will appear to have different lengths or patterns, sometimes children have difficulty identifying them. It is essential to recognize that the way a sentence or word appears in print is not necessarily the way it sounds to a child (for example, *money* may be perceived as a monosyllabic word). If possible, allow profoundly deaf children to *feel* the stimuli; if enough vibrators are available, you also should feel the speech material. In addition, try rewriting the set of sentences in an attempt to further differentiate them, and then experimentally determine if this helps the children to identify them.

practicing specific stimulus-response tasks

Although some common practice activities and listening games seem only remotely related to conversation, they can be of considerable value to auditory speech communication (Table 5–6). These exercises may be selected be-cause the teacher has had very little auditory training experience, and may want to use carefully directed preplanned activities. Another purpose for these specific tasks is to work on particular auditory problems that the child con-sistently exhibits, such as an inability to detect voiceless fricatives, to distin-guish the word *two* from the word *three*, or to answer *where* questions. The teacher may want to practice specific listening tasks during times that have been set aside especially for individual or group auditory training. Here, the intent is not so much to communicate fluently through speech, as it is to practice particular listening skills. And the teacher also may wish to use this time to simultaneously increase his or her confidence as an auditory instruc-tor and the child's confidence as a listener.

As a teacher, you may select a basic listening task to satisfy a child's needs as indicated either by your initial auditory screening (Chapter 4), or by other informally administered auditory tests. You also may choose a listening task for practice simply on the basis of repeated observations of the child's auditory behavior.

auditory detection tasks

Some children seem unable to detect any component of speech reliably through their hearing aids. Others can detect vowels and some consonants

TABLE 5–6. Some examples of specific auditory training tasks.

DETECTION

Purpose: To determine hearing aid settings, to check if the aids are working.

To attract a child's attention and orient him or her to the listening task.

To determine which sounds are available to the child.

Response: place a block/peg in one of two locations, point to yes/no pictures.

There is rarely any need to spend much time at this level, although it may be worthwhile helping the child to detect those sounds, such as fricative consonants, which are low in acoustic energy.

Example of task: Individual speech sounds, words, phrases, or sentences may be presented. The child responds "I hear it"/"I don't hear it" (Yes/No) to presence or absence of sound (silence).

Teacher: "Say what I say: 'Sheryl'."
Child: "Errol" (_____eryl)
Teacher: "Can you hear this, *yes* or *no*?: /ʃ/."

DISCRIMINATION

Purpose: to determine if the child can detect differences or similarities in two stimuli, that is, in remedial speech-perception activities. Also can be used to test perceptual difference between speech patterns, such as loud/soft and stress/no stress.

Response: Indicate similarity or difference (same/not same).

Example of task: I. Teacher: "What day comes after Thursday?"
Child: "Wednesday"

Did he or she: a) misunderstand 'before'/'after'?

or   b) misunderstand 'Tuesday'/'Thursday'?

To discover the nature of the error you may ask: "Are these the same?":

a) "What day comes *before* Thursday."
"What day comes *after* Thursday?"

or   b) "What day comes after *Thursday*?"
"What day comes after *Tuesday*?"

or   you may check discrimination at the word level by asking, "Are these the same?":
a) before/after?
b) Tuesday/Thursday?

II. Write what you said and also what the child thought you said. Ask the child to listen again. Speak ("before") and also point to one of the written forms ("after"), asking the child if what he or she heard was the *same* as the one you indicated. (Do not necessarily expect the child to rely on memory to store

TABLE 5–6. continued

or	both words/sentences while comparing them to judge their similarities or differences, as this may be too difficult.) III. This may be done with individual speech sounds also. "Are these the same?": /m/ . . . /n/; or write /m/ on the chalkboard, then say /n/, and ask the child "Are they the same?" IV. At the word level, the teacher may show the child a picture. Teacher: "What's this?" Child: "Zebra." The teacher then covers his or her mouth and says "Cat" . . . "Is that the same?" The child responds "Yes" or "No." This is a lower level task than Identification (naming the word). Although a given child may not be able to *repeat* the two items, he or she may be able to judge if the two stimuli are the same or different.

IDENTIFICATION

Purpose:	Applying labels to speech stimuli which can be discriminated; learning speech patterns.
Response:	Point to item named by the speaker, repeat stimulus, write stimulus.
Example of task:	I. Present phonemes, syllables, words, phrases, or sentences and ask the child to name/repeat them. It is preferable to choose items that relate to a recent class discussion or activity (for example bird, egg, feather, wing, nest). II. List sentences on the chalkboard; then present each one at random for identification, for example: A. Last Thursday everybody went to the park. B. (nothing; no sound). C. All the children walked in the mud. D. Frazer's shoes got wet. E. Skipper kicked his new football. It got stuck in a tree. F. Mr. Corbett growled. G. Mrs. Davis' group went back the next day to get the football out of the tree.

When writing sentences, it is a good idea to construct ones that have some relevance to the children. Try to make the sentences sufficiently different in length and/or pattern to enable all children in the group to achieve some success in identification.

When presenting an identification task, include "no sound" (the absence of sound) as a response option. This helps the child to become aware of the

TABLE 5–6. continued

possibility that he or she may hear nothing, and so can learn to indicate that the hearing aid is off, has a dead battery, or is faulty. A response of "no sound" also may indicate that the talker is too far away from the child.

COMPREHENSION

Purpose:	Understanding the meaning of a spoken stimulus. Making complex associations between sounds and events/objects, or between sounds themselves.
Reponse:	The child performs the required task or answers questions.
Examples of task:	I. *Questions*

    A. How many sisters do you have?

    B. Who won the football game last Saturday?

    C. Where's the battery tester?

II. *Instructions*

    A. Take this message to Mrs. Dowell. (Then present message with mouth covered.)

    B. Please go and get the basketball.

    C. Tell Miss Hayes to turn off her lights.

    D. Put on your coat. It's cold outside.

    E. It's time for recess. Put your books away.

    F. Draw a picture of the school bus.

III. *Cognitive tasks*

    A. *Tell me the opposite:*

       north – hot – wet

       east – fat – big

    B. *Is this the name of an animal/food/person?* cat, teacher, hamburger, doctor, pie, potato, carrot, elephant, worm, bird, man

    C. *What am I talking about? School/shopping/weather?*

       1. It rained all day last Friday.

       2. I bought a new shirt.

       3. The bell rang.

       4. All of the children are in the playground.

       5. It's nearly spring.

       6. Let's go on the train to the city.

    D. *Word associations.* What do you think of when I say:

       "kangaroo" — hop (Child A)

                   animal (Child B)

                   Skippy (Child C)

    E. *True/False* (right/wrong).

       Teacher: "It's Wednesday," or "I'm a man," or "The sun is shining."

       Child: "Yes" or "No."

but only when these are produced with a strong vocal effort. Under either of these conditions it is useful to give the child practice at the detection level of perception (Table 5–6). A detection task has several objectives: to determine if the hearing aid is working properly; to help the child learn to find this out for himself or herself; and to prepare the child for higher-level auditory activities.

Of course, we cannot actually change the child's *sensitivity* to sound. Instead, we try to increase the child's tendency to respond to weak sounds and thereby develop his or her self-confidence. Hence, another principal purpose for the detection task is to help you understand the effects of your vocal effort, your distance from the child, and your voice pitch on the child's ability to detect speech. Also, you may practice this task simply to help the child gain familiarity with the general detection procedure, so that it may be applied at other times.

As described in Chapter 4, cueing a detection task entails placing two face pictures before the child, one of which looks as if it were producing sound (Chapter 4, Figure 4–4). With repeated practice, the young child will come to realize that whenever you present that set of symbols, you also will ask him or her to say whether or not something was heard. With older children, the printed words, *YES* and *NO*, alone can be used. After repeated practice in a drill setting, you should be able to introduce a detection task abruptly, when necessary, at any time; for example, if you suspect that the child's hearing aid is not operating properly, you can quickly check with a speech detection task.

By all means, teachers should always end an auditory training session with a listening task at which the child can succeed. The intent is to maintain a positive attitude in the child. For some children, their only successful listening activity is detection of speech, so you may choose to apply detection tasks for this purpose.

You the teacher may use the same general format that was applied during auditory screening. That is, place *YES* and *NO* pictures before the child and ask him or her to point to one when you present a stimulus (sound or no sound) behind a cover. Of course, you may allow other responses as well, for variety. For example, you may ask the child to point his or her thumb up or down, push one of two buttons, place a block in one of two locations, place a peg in one of two holes, say "yes" or "no," and so forth, whenever the child does or does not hear a spoken stimulus.

Normally, you will not want to spend much time working at the detection level. The procedure is primarily applied as a check during an ongoing identification or comprehension activity when a child's auditory difficulty seems to be based on an inability to detect a phoneme, syllable, or word (for example, the word *to* in "I went *to* Marilyn's house."). You would then practice detection of that word, and perhaps others containing the same vowel (*shoe, stew, blue, do, who, new, Sue, zoo*), changing your voice level, pitch, and distance to determine the conditions under which the child *can* detect the phoneme, syllable, or word in question. In addition you should explain and demonstrate that the phoneme / u / is associated with sound, that the child can in fact detect that sound under certain conditions (incorporating low noise, short distance, loud teacher's voice, properly working hearing aid), and that he or she must *produce* the vowel with sound also, or else people with normal hearing will not be able to understand. (You may want to reverse the practice procedure so that you serve as the listener; the child presents the phoneme, syllable, or word. You indicate that you can or cannot detect the item when he or she produces it.)

auditory discrimination tasks

The primary purpose of a discrimination task is to provide remedial listening practice when a child exhibits difficulty in identifying an item. Here, you present two or more stimuli and require the child to indicate whether they sound the same or different.

Again, there are several procedures. For example, cover your mouth and say two words or phonemes in succession, gesturing to the right and left as you speak. Gesture in such a way that you establish a "place in space" for each item—the first to your right (child's left) and the second to your left (child's right). Then ask the child if they sound the *same* or *different*. For some children, you may need to ask the question differently—"Are they the *same* or *not the same?*" or, "Are they the same, *yes* or *no?*" For a young child, it may be necessary to practice first with similar and dissimilar *objects* placed in the two locations.

It is possible to present more than two items for comparison. For three items, cover your mouth and present the sound stimuli, again gesturing in such a way as to place each in a particular location in space. For example, the first spoken item may be "placed" to your right (child's left), the second in front of you (child's center), and the third to your left (child's right). Two of the items should be the same and one different (for example, / a /-/ u /-/ a /; dog-dog-cat; in the park, around the park, around the park). Then ask the child which one is different. A verbal label is not required; merely a pointing response to a particular location. This task may be a little more difficult than the two-item one because the child must listen for a longer time and remember more before responding.

In another approach, you might cover your mouth and present a continuous sound that changes in quality at random intervals. For example, this may be a sung vowel that changes in pitch (aaaaaa| aaaaaa| aaaaaaa) or quality (/ iiiiiuiiiiiii /), or a word repeated over and over, changed at particular intervals, (stop-stop-stop-stop-*top*-stop-stop). The child's task is to indicate in some way that the sound has changed, by moving his or her hand, pointing to a different symbol, or saying "now" when he or she hears a change (Figure 5–9).

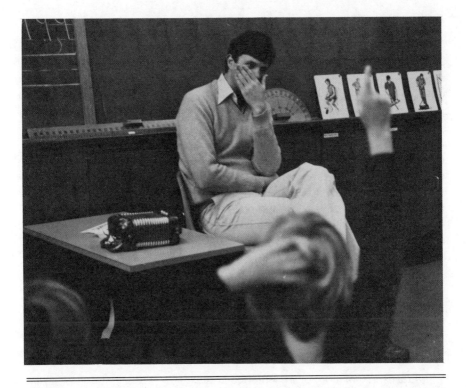

figure 5–9. A teacher presents an auditory discrimination task to a group of severely hearing-impaired children.

Further, to lessen the memory requirements, you also can present a discrimination task that requires the child to listen to only one sound stimulus at a time. First write the two phonemes, words, or phrases that the child tends to confuse. Then cover your mouth, point to one of them, and say either one of the two. Ask the child if what you said and what you pointed to are the same; he or she is to respond *yes* or *no*. Similarly, words may be presented in the form of pictures glued to cards. Pick up a picture (a blue car), cover your mouth with it, either name the picture (blue car) or say something else (red car, blue bus), then lower the picture and ask the child if what was heard is the same as the picture—whether you correctly named the picture. This is considered an entertaining game by most children. Many hearing-impaired children, who cannot correctly *identify* spoken words by pointing to pictures, are able to indicate whether the word spoken is the same as (or is different from) the name of the picture displayed.*

---

*This task can be interpreted as something like an identification task, only easier. There are only two alternatives (this picture's label or some other label), and the child need not be able to actually name the item spoken.

auditory identification tasks

Some hearing-impaired children demonstrate difficulty identifying words and/or sentences, or even placing them in correct stress-pattern categories. Others have difficulty comprehending instructions or answering questions without visible cues. Both groups may need practice in identification of speech materials of a particular type. In the first instance, the child needs identification practice to elevate performance to a higher level. In the latter case, the child has demonstrated difficulty at a high level of auditory function, and the teacher is mainly interested in discovering the source of a specific problem, for example, the word/sentence length, vocabulary content, or syntax.

The actual stimulus materials—what the teacher says to the child for identification—will depend on the child's individual auditory needs. Practice can be provided with any of the following:

voice pitch (intonation contours)

vowels, diphthongs

consonants, consonant blends

phonemes in syllable or word context

syllables in isolation or in word context

words in isolation, in phrases, or in sentence context

phrases in isolation, or in sentence context

sentences alone, or in the context of connected discourse

connected discourse (stories, songs, poems)

Typically, to establish the context for the listening activity, the teacher will write the set of items such as a list of syllables: / bi /, / bu /, / pi /, / pu /, present a set of objects to be named (bear, chair, hair, stair), or provide a picture that illustrates a set of spoken sentences (butcher shop, newsstand, park, supermarket, playground) (Table 5–6; Figure 5–10).

Then tell the child that you the teacher will say one of the items. He or she should listen, and then indicate which was presented by pointing or repeating. Usually, these tasks are presented with the mouth covered; if the child experiences difficulty, the teacher applies common remedial acoustic strategies: repetition, emphasis, speech clarification, reduction of number of alternatives, and so on. If the child makes consistent errors, such as confusions between a particular pair of items, you should note this and present a discrimination task with those items at a later time.

In consideration of the difficulties the child has with remembering long strings of syllables (as in sentences), you may choose to practice identification tasks with *words* as the speech material. Thus, initial tasks might require the child to distinguish among a small set of words with different stress patterns

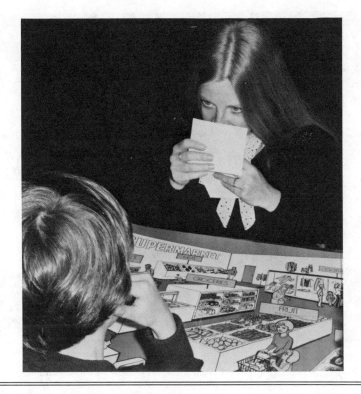

figure 5–10. An auditory identification task, in which children are asked to repeat sentences (e.g., "I went to the supermarket, and I bought some potatoes."). The teacher uses pictures to establish a context for the activity.

(for example, *cat, turtle, hot dog, ice cream cone*). Later work of this sort might require the child to identify words all having the same stress pattern, which is a more difficult task (for example, *dog, leaf, man,* or *ice cream, football, popcorn*). Even more difficult listening practice would require the child to identify words that are similar but for one or two vowels or consonants (for example, *knot, pot, pots,* or *beet, bit, bet*).

Numerous listening games can be created which depend on word or sentence identification (Figure 5–11) (Lowell & Stoner, 1960; Pollack, 1970). Such games serve several purposes. Whereas, some children respond well merely to a smile, nod, or other simple acknowledgment, others require moving a marker along a path toward a goal (indicating the endpoint of activity), or require tangible reinforcers (candy, or poker chips). Still others may be satisfied to receive the cards depicting the stimuli (child correct: child gets card; child incorrect: teacher gets card). Experience has shown that many of these enjoyable listening tasks are quite useful in maintaining a child's interest and motivation during auditory practice sessions.

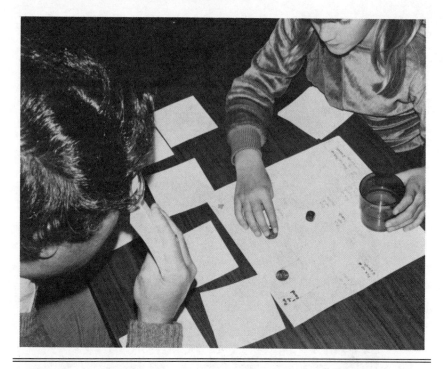

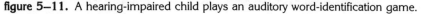

figure 5–11. A hearing-impaired child plays an auditory word-identification game.

the tracking procedure

A special method to provide identification practice with sentence-length material is the "Tracking Procedure," developed by DeFilippo and Scott (1978). It is especially useful for evaluating auditory recognition ability and for providing listening practice to hearing-impaired children. In this method, the teacher, with the mouth covered, reads brief stories (200 to 500 words each) to the child, who attempts to repeat verbatim what he or she hears. When the child makes an error, the teacher corrects repeatedly until the repetition is exact. The teacher chooses the length of each speech segment (word-by-word, phrase-by-phrase), remedial acoustic strategies (repetition, exaggeration, prompting), and when or whether to employ visible cues. Whenever the teacher uses gestures or visible articulation to clarify the speech material, this is indicated by marking the text accordingly (circles to denote words presented with audiovisual cues, brackets for words accompanied by natural gestures).

The teacher records the following measures at each practice session: 1) the total number of words contained in the story divided by the total time in minutes required to complete it (rate in words per minute); and 2) the number of words presented either with visible articulation or with gestural

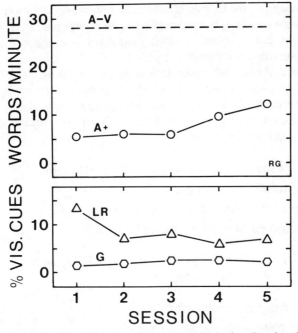

figure 5–12. Results of five listening sessions in which the "tracking" (repetition) procedure was used to provide practice in aided listening to a severely hearing-impaired teenager. The material consisted of pages from a science text. Her auditory-visual repetition rate (words/minute) is provided for reference. Some words could not be transmitted successfully unless they were accompanied by visible articulatory cues (LR) or by natural gestures (G). The percentage of words repeated under each of these conditions also is shown. (The notation "A+" indicates that communication was achieved through *auditory plus* occasional visual cues.)

prompts, divided by the total number of words in the story (proportion of words presented with visible cues). Graphs can be drawn showing how each measure changes as a function of repeated practice (Figure 5–12). The tracking procedure's aim is to maximize auditory transmission rate in words per minute, while minimizing reliance on visual cues. This is a special way of estimating a child's auditory "efficiency." In addition, you may obtain the word per minute rate for combined audiovisual conditions to estimate the child's maximum performance. You can use this comparison measure as an ultimate goal level for perception through audition alone.

auditory comprehension tasks

Some children indicate through their auditory responses that they are able to identify (repeat) requests or questions directed at them, yet are unable to demonstrate comprehension of those same sentences reliably (perform or respond as requested). Other children can comprehend spoken messages with reasonable accuracy but only when the sentences are short and of basic syntactic form. Both groups need listening practice at the comprehension level, but obviously for different reasons.

One type of comprehension task is described below. Here, the teacher places a set of pictures before the children for examination (Figure 5–13). The teacher and students then discuss them in detail. Specifically, you might display pictures depicting Olympic athletes. Cover your mouth with a card and describe one of the pictures:

1). "The Australian woman won a gold medal in diving."

2). "The Russian man is jumping."

3). "The Greek woman is throwing a javelin."

4). "Two gymnasts are flying through the air."

The child must identify which picture you describe (Figure 5–13). Then, you ask a question relating to that picture:

1). "Who came in second/third?"

2). "What color is his uniform?"

3). "How long is a javelin?"

4). "What countries do they come from?"

All of this, of course, should be done with your mouth covered. Ongoing discussion of the topic can continue, if the children are capable of the auditory (or audiovisual) activity.

There are a variety of auditory tasks that do not fit the format indicated above, but nevertheless are comprehension-related activities. These are cognitive activities, which require the child to think in terms of sound, or at least match remembered information with sound input (for example, stimulate the recall of images, develop associations, elicit complicated behavioral responses) (Table 5–6).

For these sorts of comprehension activities the child might be asked to name the opposite of the word *tall* (or *dark*, or *rough*). Or a word or sentence may be presented and the child asked to name the general class of objects/events/activities that is being presented (e.g., "table"—*furniture*; "The soccer players were very tired"—*sports*). In other tasks, the child might be asked to associate words, telling what he or she thinks of when you say, for example "rain"—*wet, puddle, mud*. Also, you might try true/false games, in which you make a statement, and the child says whether it is true or false by replying with *yes* or *no* to, for example, "There are six people in this room." Or you may tell the child a brief story (5 to 10 sentences), and then ask questions about it ("Who did Jack meet?" "How many beans did he get?"

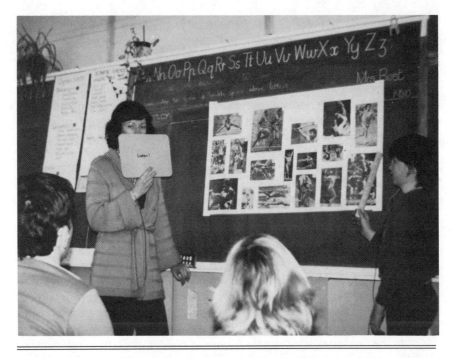

figure 5–13. An auditory comprehension task. The teacher asks questions about a set of pictures cut from newspaper articles.

What kind of beans were they?"). Of course, all of these activities would be presented with the mouth covered.

Above all, during comprehension tasks, it is extremely important to encourage the child not to verbalize at the identification level before responding. That is, do not let him or her repeat the stimulus first, wait for some indication from you that he or she is correct, and only then answer the question, perform the task, tell the opposite, and so forth. Instead, the child should be reminded to *think* before responding, to bolster self-confidence in his or her ability to do this. If the child exhibits difficulty with this emphasis, be patient, be willing to repeat, and accept errors without discomfort. Indicate that you intend to help the child achieve comprehension, that you want him or her to think in terms of sound images, and that *you* have confidence in the child's ability.

additional comments

The practice of specific stimulus-response tasks may seem to imply that auditory training should follow a quasi-developmental sequence of increasing complexity from *detection* of speech, through *discrimination, identification,* to *comprehension.* However, this third style describes only a particular instructional point of view. Numerous teachers and hearing clinicians choose instead to employ *connected speech first* (the conversational approach) in auditory training, with firm expectations for the child's comprehension. In this manner, one communicates with the hearing-impaired child in approximately the same way as one would with a normally hearing child. If difficulty in comprehension occurs, the instructor either may simplify the stimulus material, request a lower-level response from the child, or provide additional cues. Other instructors develop their own intermediate methods and strategies.

You may find it hard to accept the view that auditory training should be an experimental teaching/communication activity, without specific steps to follow. Here, you are provided with a basic rationale, structure, and direction, but what is actually said or done in the classroom is up to you. While you are first learning to do auditory training, you may feel insecure and constantly ask for advice. Please be appreciative if your more experienced colleagues do not give step-by-step instructions, but instead merely give you subtle hints to establish the conditions under which the child can succeed ("try eliminating one or two of the long sentences; or, maybe your voice is too soft."). You are more likely to remember effective auditory training methods, those that work for *you*, if you (re)create them yourself.

In the final analysis, it is not known just how or why a hearing-impaired child improves auditory perception. The sensations that a child receives through hearing aids probably do not change through auditory training. A spoken word's acoustic properties do not change very much with repeated utterances. But during the course of several days, weeks, or months, the way in which the child labels that sound pattern may change radically. For example, if you say "football" without visible cues to the child, and ask for a repetition of what you said, the child may initially tell you that he or she does not know; later, after much practice, he or she might be able to identify the final syllable, *ball.* Even later, the child might confidently label the entire word as *football,* even though his or her auditory sensation is no different from before. You have taught the child to label distorted, ambiguous acoustic cues, and just as important, you have given him or her the confidence to respond. Very often this involves simply establishing conditions in which the child can succeed and then clearly demonstrating that he or she can in fact be successful.

summary

After using the GASP! or another auditory screening test to establish the child's abilities and limitations, you will begin to guide the child's auditory development. This instruction should start at a level of performance just beyond the range of the child's present auditory capabilities. There are three general styles of auditory training that may be applied, differing in specificity, rigidity, and direction: 1) a conversational approach; 2) a moderately structured approach; and 3) practice on specific tasks. With any of these three general styles, you may apply adaptive procedures, in which the child's responses to recent speech perception activities determine the choice of tasks to be presented next. During this work, you must consider the various stimulus types (such as word or sentence) as well as response levels (such as identification or comprehension).

Auditory training need not follow a developmental plan where, for instance, you practice phoneme detection first and attempt comprehension of related sentences last. Instead, you might use the "conversational approach" during all daily conversation, and apply the "moderately structured approach" as a follow-up to each class activity. During each activity, you will note consistent errors. Later, you might provide brief periods of specific practice with difficult material. In this way, you can incorporate auditory training into conversation and instruction, rather than treat listening as a skill to be developed independent of communication.

6

some
practical suggestions

The preceding two chapters have proposed a method for quickly evaluating a hearing-impaired child's auditory capacity and then have suggested ways to improve the child's listening performance through auditory training. The three subtests of the GASP! and the auditory training exercises that follow have been applied by many teachers and hearing clinicians. These people have asked numerous relevant questions regarding the use of the materials, particularly how to apply them most effectively in their special situations. Perhaps you have similar questions. The purpose of this chapter is to anticipate and to answer them.

advantages and limitations of the GASP!

Recall that the GASP! offers the following features. It is a brief auditory screening test that can be administered in less than an hour. Most teachers can easily understand its principles and procedures. It is intended for use by teachers themselves; that is, the teacher's voice and the child's amplification system are considered essential aspects of the test. The resulting test information is directly applicable to later auditory training; the results indicate where, in general, to begin, and also which adaptive procedures are likely to be helpful. In addition, the adaptive test procedures themselves provide initial practice in auditory training for both the child and the teacher; both may be surprised at which tasks can and cannot be accomplished with only acoustic cues.

The GASP!, however, is limited in several ways. Because the test is administered by the teacher through the child's own amplification system, we cannot determine if the scores represent the child's hearing capacity; an optimal voice presenting speech through an optimal hearing aid would be required to establish that level of best performance. Also, the test is given binaurally, if the child normally wears binaural aids. Thus, each ear is not screened separately, and so we cannot judge how much each ear contributes to overall perception, or which ear is the better or "dominant" ear. Another limitation is that the GASP! samples only three of the many possible communication tasks described by the stimulus-response matrix (Chapter 4, Figure 4–1), although perhaps the school audiologist can do more extensive testing to obtain additional valuable information of this sort. Also, the audiologist can administer recorded test materials periodically to evaluate the child's auditory progress. But because the GASP! cannot be easily adapted to recorded presentation (as it is an *interactive* test), other test materials must be employed for this purpose (for example, PBF, M/J, WIPI, and TAC). (See Chapter 4.) Also, since only one form of the GASP! exists, it must be supplemented for hearing aid selection, readministering speech test materials through various hearing aids and settings to determine the optimum choice.

individual versus group auditory training

Most successful aural habilitation programs have been developed around the concept of close personal contact between the hearing therapist and the hearing-impaired child (Beebe, 1953; Grammatico, 1974, Pollack, 1970). Many teachers prefer this approach primarily because it allows them to give the child personal attention for long periods of time—devoting as much time as is required to solve a particular listening problem without worry about interruptions from classroom schedules or from other children. Moreover, it may be easier to plan auditory training sessions; materials and activities can be constructed and assembled specifically for the individual child's interest and needs. With only one child in the room with the instructor, the surrounding environment usually will be quiet and relatively free of distractions. During these personal sessions, it usually is easy to attract and maintain one child's attention, because he or she is just across the table, within arm's reach. At this distance, the signal-to-noise ratio is improved, that is, the quality of the amplified speech signal that the child receives is enhanced (Figure 6–1). This close proximity also allows the teacher to manipulate objects near the child as well as to guide the child in making particular responses. In a single session with an individual child, it may be possible to solve perplexing auditory problems that otherwise might take weeks to diagnose and/or resolve.

In contrast, numerous teachers, clinics, and schools prefer to instruct children in groups rather than as individuals. What are the reasons? First, providing individual instruction for long periods of time is an expensive way

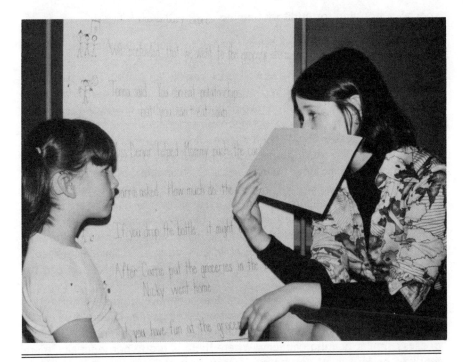

figure 6–1. A teacher provides special practice in listening (sentence identification) to a single child.

to teach, and may be beyond the financial range of most public-supported institutions. But there are other reasons that have been suggested by teachers themselves. Intensive *individual* instruction can be exhausting for both the teacher and the child. While working in a *group*, a child learns a sense of cooperation, the importance of keeping quiet while someone else is listening, and how to behave socially during an interactive, group conversation (for example, how to take turns talking). In a discussion group, the children can help one another, by offering suggestions, prompts, strategies, or encouragement that might not be as motivating if provided by the teacher alone. Also, a group setting can simplify interactive teaching in some situations; during a breakdown in communication, the teacher may have more options, such as requesting a response from another child if persistent difficulty occurs. (If not applied carefully, however, this strategy can lead to neglect of children with poorer hearing.) Actually, most teachers accept a compromise between group and individual instruction, and try to arrange auditory training within *small groups* of two or three children. This compromise allows them either to provide individual attention to each child, or to conduct an interactive conversation if they desire. It also produces reasonable quiet and lack of distraction during the session.

special regrouping for auditory training

In most schools and classes for the hearing impaired, learning groups are formed on the basis of the children's age and language performance (receptive language and reading as well as expressive language). Typically, when administrators separate children on this basis, they are not specifically concerned with the way in which a given hearing-impaired child uses his or her sensory systems to obtain speech (spoken language) information. For this reason, many classes contain hearing-impaired children who differ widely in auditory ability. This arrangement can make it very difficult for the teacher to conduct group auditory training sessions, because certain children may hear considerably better than others; some children will be limited to tactile perception of sound patterns (Figure 6–2), while others will be able to understand almost everything the teacher says by listening alone. Consequently, many teachers have suggested re-forming classes (for auditory training purposes at least) on the basis of the children's *auditory* abilities. The results from the GASP! can help determine which children should be grouped together.

In connection with this viewpoint, teachers have suggested numerous reasons to form special groups for auditory training. First, it should be easier to develop efficient auditory training strategies if all the children in the class possess similar hearing capacity. Where there is group homogeneity, there tends to be less overt competition among the children in terms of whose hearing is "best," and, so, less disruptive behavior emerges from those whose hearing is "poorest." In addition, the teacher would have the opportunity to develop personal auditory training skills without concern for other pressures, such as maintaining a balance of "easy" and "difficult" listening activities for children with hearing capacities ranging from poor to good. Also, if a newly formed homogeneous group meets at special times, say, once per day, then the instructor can concentrate attention on improving the hearing abilities of the children without constantly worrying about the information content of the spoken messages. New material can be introduced outside of the auditory training period through auditory-*visual* presentation, in order to reinforce and maximize transmission of that information.

On the other hand, regrouping of children requires that the teachers and the school administrators all contribute considerable out-of-class time for planning, scheduling, and review, involving careful examination of speech perception screening scores as well as personal observations. The entire staff must be cooperative and flexible. They may find it difficult, if not impossible, to form a reasonable number of homogeneous groups because few of the available children are in fact similar to one another.* Also, a particular young

---

*In forming groups, you must take into consideration factors other than the child's hearing capacity, such as age, general behavior, maturity, visual ability, language level, compatibility with other children, compatibility with particular teachers, and so on.

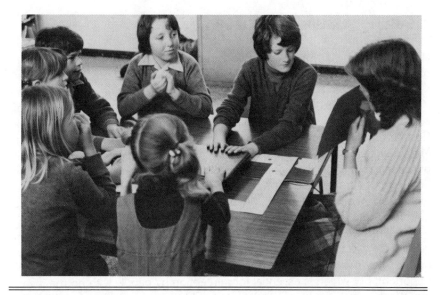

figure 6–2. A teacher provides special instruction to a group of six profoundly hearing-impaired children brought together daily in order to practice vibrotactile perception of speech.

child may find it emotionally upsetting to be assigned to an unfamiliar teacher for auditory training, after having formed a strong attachment to the regular teacher. Perhaps the most perplexing problem is that the auditory training teacher may have difficulty constructing relevant listening materials or tasks for the group because of incomplete knowledge of the activities that each child experiences with his or her regular class. This sometimes results in teacher and children practicing with mutually uninteresting material. And, after regrouping, there may be a tendency for each regular teacher to feel that all necessary auditory training is provided by the special auditory training teacher during that part of the day, and that there is little need to direct much effort to providing listening practice at other times throughout the day.

Obviously, both positive and negative arguments are valid. When a school division chooses *not* to regroup, and if listening practice is *not* scheduled for a special time of day, some teachers may neglect to incorporate auditory training into any of their daily activities. This can happen if they are new teachers, with little confidence, and are primarily concerned with managing classroom behavior and providing content information to the children. On the other hand, if regrouping is chosen as the strategy, teachers may tend to develop auditory training expertise only with a particular group (type) of children. Hence, if groups are formed, it might be worthwhile to rotate them so that each teacher develops a variety of auditory training skills that can be incorporated into each one's homeroom at other times of the day. Each school, class, or clinic would have to develop its own arrangement, according to the children and staff personnel available.

"auditory" training with a vibrator

Using a hand-held vibrator has been suggested either for extended testing of a profoundly hearing-impaired child's pattern perception skills (Chapter 4) or for developing the child's abilities in speech perception and production (Chapters 5, 7, and 9). Vibrotactile transducers have been used as part of auditory training in several established educational programs (Asp, 1973; Connors & McPherson, 1979; Guberina, 1964; Schulte, 1978) (Figure 6–3). Many teachers unfamiliar with the vibratory training concept frequently ask questions regarding the application of this special type of device, such as how can a vibrator help a profoundly deaf child; and how should the audiologist or teacher determine whether the child needs to use a vibrotactile aid rather than a more conventional hearing aid?

There are several important reasons for providing vibrotactile speech cues to a profoundly hearing-impaired child. First, it helps develop an awareness of the *acoustic* nature of speech, which the child may consider unimportant, but which is essential for perception by people with normal hearing. Within a few weeks of practice it should be apparent that the child can use a tactile aid to distinguish spoken words and sentences with different

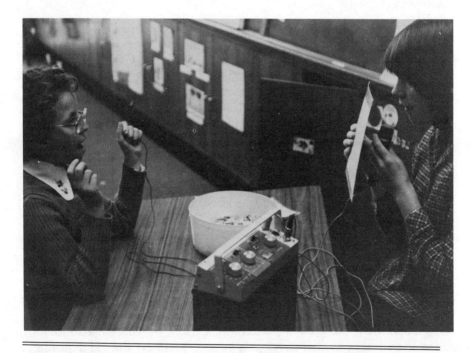

figure 6–3. A teacher gives a child practice in receiving speech patterns through a hand-held vibrator.

TABLE 6–1. Sounds detected by a group of children who used a portable vibrator during an out-of-school excursion.

trams (streetcars)
trucks
motorbikes
buses
dogs barking
children hopping as they play hopscotch
cars
the pump motor at the swimming pool
children banging on a street sign
a man jumping on wood in a truck
a woman starting her car
an airplane flying overhead
a girl laughing
the water from a water fountain falling in the sink
the motor in the boiler room
Mr. Fisher pushing a wheelbarrow on concrete
a boy talking
a door slamming
birds pecking food on a tin
an alarm clock ringing

stress patterns. Also, tactile cues can help the child lipread, by removing some of the ambiguity in a speaker's visible articulation (Erber, 1972b, 1979d). Most important, unless the child receives the acoustic component of speech while lipreading, he or she is likely to develop an unnatural concept of spoken language as a silent articulatory event; this impoverished view may be reflected in the quality of his or her own speech (for example, inappropriate or poorly timed voicing). Tactile cues allow the child to monitor his or her speech, in general, by providing an indication of its overall loudness, rate, and rhythm, and, in particular, by helping the child minimize certain articulatory deviations such as extreme burst intensity in final plosives, such as / p / in the word *lip* (Schulte, 1978).

In addition, use of a vibrator can help the profoundly hearing-impaired child develop an appreciation for the sounds of the world around him (Plant, 1979). This includes acquiring the ability to detect and identify natural environmental sounds—airplanes flying overhead—as well as sounds that can be directly relevant to the child's welfare—someone's voice, or a car approaching (Table 6–1).

In general, therefore, it is advisable to provide a child with speech stimulation through a vibrator if hearing loss is so extreme that a conventional hearing aid cannot provide sufficient acoustic power to reliably elicit even detection responses without discomfort or feedback squeal. In these cases, of course, the audiologist also must make an effort to obtain an aid (*acoustic amplifier*) that can present appropriate sound levels to the child's *ear* without acoustic feedback. At the same time you, the teacher, must consistently speak closely enough to the microphone to provide an adequate level of sound stimulation to the child (through whatever device he or she is using).

Continued use of a vibrator may not be necessary if a sufficiently powerful acoustic (hearing) aid can be obtained for the child. But in some cases, such as those involving meningitis or chronic otitis media, the child's lack of sensitivity to acoustic input at the ear is not likely to be resolved, and you should provide sound patterns to the child by whatever means possible. For example, you can use a vibrator connected to a wired or portable amplifier. Ideally, you would employ the device throughout the school day, whenever the child needs to receive sound to enhance communication. Several commercial units are currently available (the Mono- or Poly-Fonator manufactured by Siemens), but a technician can easily construct a vibrotactile aid from a microphone, amplifier, and bone-conduction transducer (for example, the Radioear B-71 made by Radioear Corporation) (Plant, 1979). The child and teacher should experiment with various body receptors, although the fingers, hands, and wrist seem to be the most sensitive locations (Figure 6–2 and 6–3) despite the fact that the child must use his or her hands for writing and overall manipulation. Usually it is recommended that the *teacher* also obtain a considerable amount of experience feeling speech through the vibrotactile system to be used, in order to develop an understanding of which stimuli are and are not likely to be distinguishable tactually (Erber, 1978, 1979d; Erber & Zeiser, 1974; Zeiser & Erber, 1977). In the ideal situation, both you and the child should feel a vibrator concurrently during instruction, so that you will be constantly aware of the nature of the patterns that your voice is producing.

You can implement vibratory training in much the same way as auditory training, recognizing that the child will perceive (and learn to interpret) mainly *intensity patterns* through his or her skin. Thus, a child is not likely to be able to *identify* your spoken words or sentences tactually unless you restrict the set and provide considerable practice (Figure 6–4). It may be more reasonable to direct the child's attention to generalizable aspects of speech patterns, such as duration, intensity, "roughness", syllable rate, etc. (Chapter 2, Figure 2–9 and, Chapter 9, Figure 9–1).

If a portable vibrotactile aid is available (Boothroyd, 1972; Connors & McPherson, 1979; Plant, 1979) then the child can use the device continually throughout the day, both in and out of class. If a portable amplifier cannot be obtained, however, both you and the audiologist should help the child make the transfer from the stronger vibrotactile speech patterns received from a wired classroom vibrator to the less prominent intensity pattern possibly received through his or her personal, portable hearing aid(s). One way to accomplish this transfer is to hold the vibrator against the hearing aid

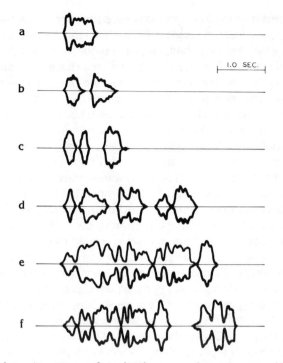

figure 6—4. Intensity patterns of words, phrases, and sentences used in a vibrotactile identification exercise with profoundly hearing-impaired children (similar to examples given in Chapter 5, Tables 5–3 and 5–6): a) "banana," b) "ice cream," c) "chocolate syrup," d) "whipped cream, some nuts, and a cherry," e) "A little girl wanted to make a banana split," and f) "After the girl made the banana split, she ate it."

receiver or earmold at the child's ear, gradually attenuating the level of the speech signal to the vibrator, as the child attends to the output of the hearing aid.

The ultimate contribution that tactile experience with speech patterns can make to a hearing-impaired child's communication development remains unknown. As teachers continue to gain experience in tactile training, we are gradually accumulating the knowledge to guide us.

auditory versus auditory-visual instruction

Both laboratory research and clinical experience have shown that nearly all hearing-impaired people understand speech optimally when they are able to lipread while listening through their hearing aids (Erber, 1975). Thus, when communication of important information is the object of speech (at home or in the classroom), simultaneous attention to acoustic and optical inputs is the best method to insure accurate perception of the message. For example, if a parent wants to explain, for the first time, how to plant pumpkin seeds to a hearing-impaired child, he or she probably should do so through auditory-visual communication so that the child can have the best opportunity to comprehend the complicated instructions and new vocabulary.

When the goal, however, is to provide special practice for the child in developing perceptual skills important for speech communication, then concentrated effort in each sensory mode alone can be very beneficial. This is true even though most hearing-impaired people usually combine audition and vision when they communicate and even though the acoustic input itself is insufficient for comprehension by many with serious hearing impairments. In fact, it often will be easier to direct the hearing-impaired child's attention to particular acoustic characteristics of words or phrases, if you cover your mouth and present the items in isolation from the visible speech cues that normally accompany them. And, of course, a child must practice auditory-only perception if he or she wishes to improve communication by telephone.

The question of whether to use an auditory-only or an auditory-visual approach becomes difficult when considering auditory training in the education of the hearing-impaired infant or very young child. It is clear that all children must learn to make many auditory-visual associations during their development, such as a dog and the sound of barking or a firetruck and the sound of its siren, with repeated reinforcement of these associations so that everyday sounds become meaningful. Our present concern is whether to exclude vision during *speech* communication with the child (the unisensory approach) or whether to allow the child to lipread while listening to your voice (the multisensory approach). Those who advocate a unisensory method feel that if an infant with a serious hearing impairment is encouraged to use vision to attend to faces, he or she may never bother to attend to, and learn to use, those acoustic cues that are perceptually difficult. Those who support a multisensory approach feel that the child should be allowed to develop a bisensory process of audition and vision for communication, using whatever speech information is accessible in each modality.

A direct comparison between unisensory and multisensory approaches is difficult because strict application of each instructional method rarely is made. Teachers who prefer auditory-alone procedures tend to resort to auditory-visual input whenever a child has difficulty perceiving speech acoustically, while the auditory-visual advocates often provide special listening activities when confident of the child's auditory success.

It seems sensible to consciously adopt an experimental attitude and a degree of flexibility toward the use of auditory-only communication (or an "adaptive" approach)—that is, providing listening opportunities during the day whenever possible and requiring the child to listen to a part of everything you say. If, however, listening alone for long periods is too difficult for the child, or interferes with communication, be willing to modify your acoustic approach by providing a greater proportion of visible cues. On the other hand, try speaking with your mouth covered a greater proportion of the time if you discover that the child can understand nearly everything by listening alone.

reminders

noise annoys

Children gain the most benefit from auditory training when they practice listening in a quiet place. Children with hearing impairments need quiet environments for adequate communication. The greater the child's hearing impairment, the quieter the listening environment must be. Children can be calm, quiet, and cooperative, or they can be noisy and disruptive, contributing most of the unwanted sound in a classroom. Children's noise levels will fluctuate considerably as a function of class grouping and time of day.

How can you encourage hearing-impaired children to work quietly? Some are not aware of how loud or disruptive they can be. You must show them how to monitor their own voice levels and how to keep themselves quiet. In addition, you can: provide meaningful tasks to keep children quietly busy; devise methods for withdrawing individuals for a quiet conversation; develop behavior management techniques to personally control the group; and encourage communicative cooperation.

In addition, you should recognize that most objects that a child might bring into the room (ruler, book, pen) will make noise if pounded or thumped against a chair or table, and so they may serve as distractors. Ask the children to place their possessions in another part of the room when they enter. Ask them to help you keep the room quiet!

do not plan too far ahead

There is no need to follow a prepared lesson plan closely. If you discover in the middle of an auditory training session that what you have prepared is too easy or too difficult for the children, change the activity to suit their abilities. For example, if you had planned a word identification task with pictures of animals, and it is too *easy* for the children, try asking them comprehension questions about the animals, or the zoo, or their pets. If the task is too *difficult*, try working with a more limited set, include words with very different stress patterns, or present a task at the discrimination level.

It is probably not worth the trouble to prepare elaborate teaching materials before an auditory training session. If the preparation time is great relative to the duration of the stimulus-response activity itself (for example, identifying a word), then the preparation has been too extensive. Rather than prepare complicated pictures, cutouts, objects, and so forth, try simply writing or drawing on the chalkboard instead (or scratch in the dirt with a sharp stick).

keep a level head

Do not spend a lot of time on low-level auditory tasks, such as *detection* of speech sounds, if the children are capable of performing at a much higher level, such as identification of sentences. Try to give children the most practice at the highest level of which they are capable. Try higher level tasks occasionally to challenge them. Use lower level tasks primarily as remedial activities when you are not sure why a child has failed to respond correctly. You also may introduce easy listening activities as a change of pace during intensive instruction, or to allow the child merely to experience success without excessive effort.

sound advice

Do not give up on auditory communication too soon. If you ask a question with your mouth covered, and the child cannot answer it, do not uncover your mouth immediately. Try again, either through simple repetition, with emphasis on a particular word, or with supplementary verbal prompts. You may eventually let the child lipread certain key words, but try several times with your mouth covered before providing visible articulation.

cooperative listening

Try to avoid competitive group listening games where one child's hearing ability is set against another's. That is, do not present an acoustic stimulus to the group and then ask who knows the answer. Usually, the result will be enthusiastic screaming. Instead, ask one child at a time to sit beside you in front of the class (alternatives or pictorial material on the chalkboard) and then present the task directly as the others watch. Each time, ask the others if the child's response is correct. Give each child a turn during the session. This method avoids a competitive atmosphere and also brings the chosen child close to you for careful listening.

hail and farewell!

Try to vary listening activities both between and within sessions, so that the children (and you) remain interested and attentive. You may be able to relate all of the activities to a special theme, for example, animals, weather, or favorite foods. In addition:

1). Begin with a brief *introductory* activity to orient the children to listening—something easy such as sound detection or word naming.

2). Present a *main* activity in which you try something new or difficult. Take chances and challenge the children to perform auditory tasks that may be unfamiliar to them, for example, remembering three related verbal instructions, telling the opposites of words, or answering comprehension questions following a story.

3). Conclude with a brief *departure* activity presenting a previously practiced auditory task to bolster the children's confidence in their listening abilities. For example, say "Billy, you may go to lunch" or, "Belinda, please pick up your books!"

Remember, always try to end each auditory training session with a task at which each child can succeed. The purpose is to maintain a positive attitude toward listening. Use activities that you have tried before and which each child likes to do.

summary

We have presented some practical suggestions for auditory evaluation and training. The GASP! is a rapid screening test, whose results can guide later auditory training. Because of its lack of reliability, however, other auditory tests also should be administered annually to chart the child's progress. In addition, providing auditory training to small groups of children, homogeneous in hearing capacity is suggested. It may be desirable to form special auditory training groups that meet regularly, perhaps daily, while not limiting a child's listening practice to these sessions alone. Instead, auditory experiences should be provided throughout the day as part of classroom instruction and verbal communication. For a child with a profound hearing impairment, who seems able to perceive only intensity patterns of speech through his or her hearing aid(s), a vibrotactile transducer (such as a "bone" vibrator) may enable you to provide a prominent speech signal. Further, the teacher should provide a convenient balance between *auditory-visual* instruction (to introduce new concepts and vocabulary) and *auditory* practice (to develop a child's listening abilities). And finally, the effectiveness of auditory training can be increased by maintaining an atmosphere of flexibility, creativity, and cooperation. It is important to keep the child's needs, interests, abilities, and limitations in mind while communicating, in order to achieve maximum success and thus to derive maximum pleasure—for both teacher and child—from auditory development.

7

tape-card recordings

Hearing-impaired children differ in their ability to interpret the amplified sounds of speech. In some cases, a child's auditory perceptual system may be so seriously limited that speech can be analyzed only as gross patterns (Chapter 2). In other instances the quality or quantity of a child's daily auditory experiences may be the limiting factor affecting development; a noisy home or school environment may make it difficult for the hearing-impaired child to learn language through his or her ears (Borrild, 1978; Watson, 1964). Group methods of auditory training as commonly used in the classroom may not be sufficient in these cases. Instead, a more carefully controlled *individual* approach may be necessary to help each child acquire an awareness of the relevant components of speech and develop auditory identification and comprehension skills.

need for individual practice in listening

Specific individual practice in perceiving speech is considered desirable for many hearing-impaired children (Beebe, 1953; Doehring, 1968; Grammatico, 1974; Pollack, 1970). The following reasons are given: 1) children who are performing at different auditory skill levels require materials that differ in complexity; 2) children who differ in auditory learning ability require a different number of trials or repetitions to reach a criterion level of performance; 3) children are known to differ in their ability to make decisions and respond

121

appropriately to auditory tasks; and 4) children may require different types or amounts of reinforcement to maintain their attention or motivation. Carefully planned and directed personalized listening activities, however, typically require the full-time involvement of a teacher or parent, whose busy schedule may not allow for an adequate portion of time working with an individual child. Ideally, a hearing specialist, an assistant, or a teacher-aide would be available to direct attention to each child according to his or her particular listening needs.

self-instruction devices

As a supplement to individual instruction, several investigators have designed and constructed automated devices which provide individualized listening practice to hearing-impaired children without requiring a large amount of direct teacher or parent participation (Boothroyd, 1972; Doehring, 1968; Ling & Doehring, 1969; Risberg & Spens, 1967). These systems are comparable to one another, employing both a two-channel tape recorder to play back speech items and control tones, and an automated slide projector to present visible patterns (such as pictures or words) that are to be associated with the acoustic stimuli. When the child pushes a response button, the apparatus indicates his or her correct or incorrect choice.

Although automated instruction devices of this sort have been shown to be effective in improving children's auditory perception, all have similar limitations. First, they are relatively expensive in their present form, requiring a stereo tape recorder and an automatic slide projector, as well as special electronic circuitry. Second, the instructional programs usually are "linear"— the acoustic stimuli follow one another in the order in which they were recorded on tape. Reordering the sounds usually requires tape dubbing and/ or splicing, which involves considerable time and effort. Third, recording the speech and operating the apparatus both require some sophistication with electromechanical equipment, and many teachers cannot use the device without special instruction. And fourth, it is a time-consuming process for someone to construct the optical stimuli, which must be photographed and developed into slides. For all of these reasons, apparatus of this sort has not been widely used by teachers of the hearing impaired.

audio tape-card apparatus

The desire to employ relatively inexpensive and uncomplicated apparatus for individual instruction has led to the application of special record-playback machines that rely on audio tape-cards to present stimuli (Erber, 1976; Sims, 1978) (Figure 7–1). This apparatus permits recording and playback from a short strip of magnetic tape bonded to a stiff card. The card is mechanically

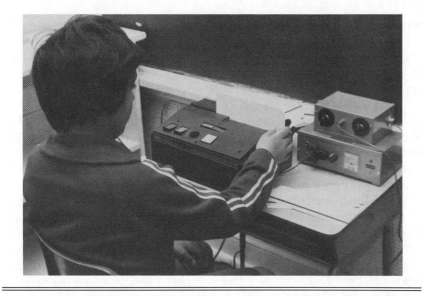

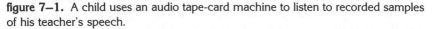

figure 7–1. A child uses an audio tape-card machine to listen to recorded samples of his teacher's speech.

transported through a narrow groove, past a two-channel magnetic recording head. An electrical switch is used to select a channel as input to the single amplifier. An output jack, intended primarily for earphones, also allows connection to a VU meter, attenuators, miniature hearing-aid receivers, bone vibrators, or other monitoring devices or transducers.

Although the present-day audio tape-card machine cannot be considered a high fidelity device, it nevertheless has been employed in auditory training because it meets the following criteria: 1) it is simple to operate by both teachers and young hearing-impaired children; 2) it presents both acoustic and optical stimuli (written, drawn on, or attached to the card) that can be constructed easily by the teacher or an assistant; 3) it permits reordering or randomizing of sound stimuli simply by shuffling the tape-cards; 4) it clearly indicates the passage of time by the visible movement of a tape-card through the machine; 5) it makes speech tangible, in that a child can manipulate and reorder the tape-cards on which the spoken items are recorded; 6) it allows discrete auditory observation intervals, defined for the child through card notching (to be described later); and 7) it is inexpensive, relative to many other auditory self-instruction devices.

The chief drawback of most current apparatus is that minor instability can occur in the tape-card transport mechanism, resulting in audible jitter and frequency shifts. This problem can be minimized by periodically cleaning the recording head and rollers with alcohol and inspecting the cards for physical damage.

modifications and accessories for tape-card machines

Most commercial tape-card machines, by themselves, are inadequate auditory training devices. Hence, they must be modified slightly to make them appropriate for use with hearing-impaired children.

For example, to record speech signals with little background noise, an external microphone is recommended (Figure 7–2). (If you use the built-in microphone instead, the recordings will usually contain audible motor rumble and hum, transmitted to the microphone through the supporting case of the machine.) Also, you can make higher-quality recordings of your speech by holding the external microphone near your mouth.

The loudspeaker built into the tape-card machine is not recommended for playback to hearing-impaired children for these reasons: it will contribute its own distortion, even at low output levels; and its sound output will mix with room noise and reflected signals (echo, or reverberant sound) before reaching the child. Instead, many instructors try to deliver the acoustic output of the machine directly to the hearing-impaired child. One simple method is to plug a set of earphones into the output jack, using monaural or stereo earphones, as specified by the machine's manufacturer (Figure 7–3a). However, the earphones supplied by most manufacturers are not recommended for this purpose since they tend to be of poor quality. Audiometric earphones with comfortable cushions, miniature hearing aid receivers (that snap into earmolds) connected to a custom-made cord, or a set of high-quality stereo earphones (with an appropriate electrical adapter plug to convert to monaural if necessary) are better choices. Even if you use earphones directly like this, the acoustic output level may be inadequately low for some severely or profoundly hearing-impaired children. If so, a local technician should be contacted to perform internal modification of the playback amplifier to boost the output sufficiently (Erber, 1976).

Another method for linking the child more directly to the audiotape-card machine is to plug a pair of miniature magnetic induction loops ("mini-loops") into the output jack (Sims, 1978). These devices convert the recorded signal to current changes in coils of wire (loops) which produce electromagnetic variations in the vicinity of the loops. Place these small coils beside the child's own hearing aid(s), with perhaps Velcro, and switch the aid(s) to the "T" (telecoil) position. The electromagnetic variations around the loop

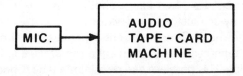

figure 7–2. An external microphone may be connected to an audio tape-card machine to maximize the fidelity of the recording by minimizing motor rumble and hum.

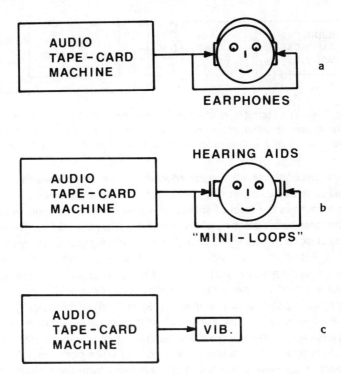

figure 7–3. A variety of output transducers may be connected directly to an audio tape-card machine, to eliminate the disruptive effects of room noise and reverberation that often occur when the built-in loudspeaker is used: earphones (a); "mini-loops" and hearing aids (b); and vibrator (c).

are detected by the telecoil, transferred to the hearing aid amplifier, and subsequently converted to sound by the hearing aid earphone (Figure 7–3b). This method serves not only to bypass the loudspeaker and thus the room environment, but allows the child to continue listening through his or her personal amplification system, which should provide sufficient gain and appropriate frequency response, if it has been selected and adjusted correctly.

For profoundly deaf children, a (bone-conduction) vibrator may be plugged directly into the "earphone" output jack. Many tape-card machines have sufficient electrical power to operate this sort of transducer. The child holds the vibrator in his or her hand or between the forefinger and thumb and feels the intensity patterns of the speech played back from the tape-cards (Erber, 1978) (Figure 7–3c).

A special output accessory box may be constructed containing a VU meter for monitoring playback level, separate attenuators (for example, 15 ohm, 3 dB step, 30 dB range) for right and left ears, right and left earphone output jacks, and a vibrator output jack (Figure 7–4). Use of an attenuator

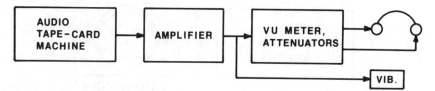

figure 7–4. The output level of an audio tape-card machine can be increased by a supplementary amplifier, monitored on a VU meter, and then controlled with attenuators. The signal is delivered to the child through earphones or a vibrator.

box like this converts a tape-card machine into a basic "speech audiometer" as well as a useful auditory training device. Once the system is calibrated, you can control the level of sound delivered to each ear independently and specify these levels in terms of dB sound pressure level (SPL). The attenuator box as described, however, provides no amplification of its own. Thus, to use this sort of accessory adequately, with severely and profoundly hearing-impaired children, it may be necessary for a technician to increase the output of the tape-card machine either by modifying its amplifier or by attaching an external supplementary amplifier (Figure 7–4) (Erber, 1976).

A mixer-amplifier, as shown below, is recommended as a very practical wired desk-top system for auditory training with a tape-card machine (Figure 7–5). This system allows presentation of live voice both from the child and the teacher, as well as recorded speech from tape-cards. Speech can be delivered to the child through earphones or through a vibrator at levels that you can monitor, attenuate in dB steps, and specify in dB SPL. This sort of custom-built apparatus is optimal for auditory training, but you can use other similar equipment as well—a public address mixer/amplifier, any good quality amplifier with multiple inputs, or perhaps a wired auditory training amplifier. Each requires an auxiliary (high-level) input jack to connect with the tape-

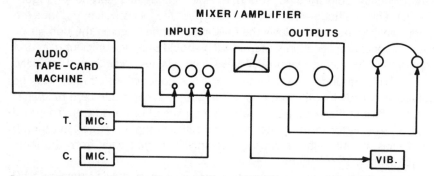

figure 7–5. An audio tape-card machine (recorded speech items) and two microphones (teacher's/child's live voice) can be used as inputs to a mixer/amplifier. Output signals are monitored, controlled, and delivered to the child through earphones or a vibrator. This arrangement provides a very flexible system for auditory training.

card playback machine. A mixer/amplifier is best, as it offers presentation of either live or recorded speech, and allows the instructor to alternate them if desired.

examples of listening activities

In individualized auditory training with a tape-card machine, each child's practice materials are prepared according to his or her specific needs (Chapter 4). General tape-card formats have been designed for each level of response difficulty (Erber, 1976). You may adapt these as needed to each type of speech material that you use. Although presenting *speech* primarily, you may desire to record and play back environmental sounds as well. Some examples of audio tape-card tasks appropriate for each level of response difficulty are outlined briefly in Table 7–1. Here, diagrams specify the appearance of the cards, that is, how (or if) you should notch* them, and what to write and record on them. A typical listening/learning program of this sort might include between 10 and 50 cards. The variety of stimuli constructed at each response level is limited only by the length of a tape-card (a 23 cm card is equal to about 3.5 seconds)** and by the teacher's creativity.

auditory detection tasks

Detection tasks are simply two-alternative forced-choice procedures in which the child sorts cards or card segments into sound or no-sound categories. For example, if you the teacher feel that a child needs practice detecting his name (*Robert*), you might record "Robert" on ten cards and mix these with ten blank cards. You would ask the child to listen to each card in turn, and to decide whether a speech stimulus is present or not, then placing the card accordingly into the *YES* box ("I hear something.") or the *NO* box ("I don't hear anything."). It may be helpful to record the "Robert" cards in Robert's presence, so that he understands what message is contained on those cards that produce an acoustic speech stimulus. (See Table 7–2A for a more detailed procedure.)

---

*"Notching" a card along the bottom edge with a 1 cm wide by 2 cm high opening (cut through the magnetic tape strip) causes the card to stop moving as the notch passes the roller/recording head assembly. Stopping the card in this way helps the child to separate the listening task into distinct observation intervals.

**It is not a good idea to record and play back cards at the special half speed available on some tape-card machines. This slow rate further diminishes the quality of the recorded sound.

TABLE 7–1. Examples of general audio tape-card formats for individual listening practice. Tasks of this sort may be applied as part of auditory training at each response level.

I. Detection (presence/absence of sound)

a. [stimulus] [(blank)]   b. [1 | 2]

T: Record stimulus cards and mix with equal number blank cards.	T: Record stimulus on either first *or* second half of card.
C: Listen: place card in *YES* or *NO* box.	C: Listen; place card in *1* or *2* box.

II. Discrimination (same/different)

a. [1 | 2]   b. [ref.] [stim.]

T: Record the two segments either with same or different stimuli.	T: Record target stimulus on reference card; record various stimuli, including target, on other cards.
C: Listen: place card in *SAME* or *DIFFERENT* box.	C: Listen; compare each stimulus card with reference; place in *SAME* or *DIFFERENT* box.

III. Identification, recognition (labeling)

a. [1. ~~~~ 2. ~~~~ 3. ~~~~ 4. ~~~~]   b. [   ]

T: Record stimulus on card; write alternatives on front of card, write correct response on back of card or in answer book.	T: Record categorical stimulus: e.g., pause/no pause in sentence; male/female talker.
C: Listen; write response; turn card over or look in answer book for correct response.	C: Listen; place card into appropriately labeled box.

IV. Comprehension (understanding meaning)

a. [   ]   b. [   ]

T: Record question on card; write correct answer on back of card or in answer book.	T: Record instruction on card; describe correct behavior in answer book.
C: Listen; write response; turn card over or look in answer book for correct response.	C: Listen; perform task as specified; consult answer book for description of correct response.

TABLE 7–2. Detailed auditory training procedures. Three examples are given in detail. You can use the first, a multiple choice procedure, both for detection and identification tasks. The second and third, related to discrimination and comprehension, respectively, are more specific in intent.

Example A. General purpose: to teach hearing-impaired children to label acoustic speech stimuli. Hypothetical problem: a profoundly hearing-impaired child cannot distinguish reliably between silence, monosyllabic words, and spondees.

1. Before the child arrives, sort prerecorded cards into separate categories and place them in boxes labeled appropriately (e.g., (nothing),—,— —).
2. The child wears earphones, or holds a vibrator, or both. Either you or the child should adjust the volume to the preferred (or "best") setting.
3. Show the labels on the boxes to the child. Indicate through speech and/ or gestures that all of the tape-cards in a given box belong to the same category as that depicted on the box.
4. Take a card set from one box and spread the cards for the child. He or she picks one, listens to it, and returns it to the appropriate box. (It is best to start with the box containing cards with the most prominent acoustic pattern.) Do this several times for each set of cards. While playing each card, remind the child which box (stimulus category) it came from, pointing to the drawn symbol on the appropriate box as the card is being played. The object is to show the child that all of the stimulus cards found in each box are members of a particular category, and that they belong in that box.
5. Take one card from each box (one from each stimulus category), show the child that you intend to mix them, and then do it (slowly). Then, select one card at random from this small "deck," request the child to listen to it and to place it in the appropriate box. (a) Repeat this procedure without replacing the played cards in the small deck. When only one unplayed card remains, ask the child to predict its category before listening to it. (b) Repeat this procedure, but replace the cards in the small deck after the child has listened to each one and identified its category. This task is more difficult than that in (a) because the probability of a correct response by chance (guessing) remains constant for each successive card.
6. Take each entire set of cards out of its respective box and place these sets side-by-side on the table, showing the child where each group of stimuli came from. Then, pick up all of the card sets, show the child that you intend to mix *all* of the cards, and then do it (slowly). Play this large deck of cards to the child one at a time (in random order). Ask him or her to identify each stimulus in turn and place it in the appropriate box. As the child performs this task, acknowledge correct responses.

Sometimes, rather than giving only verbal or gestural reinforcement, it is helpful to draw the correct symbol on the back of each card, to be shown to the child on completion of each (correct or incorrect) response.

During all of these steps, it is important that the child carefully attend to your instructions and/or gestures. You should be confident that a child understands each step in the procedure before advancing to the next one.

Example B. General purpose: to teach hearing-impaired children to perceive

TABLE 7–2. continued

fine distinctions between words. Hypothetical problem: a severely hearing-impaired child exhibits difficulty in identifying the word *monkey;* he frequently identifies it as *money, Monday,* and so on.

1. Prerecord a set of tape-cards including: one target card (*monkey*), with an appropriate picture and label attached; a group of stimulus cards containing the same word, but no picture; a group of cards containing words which the child frequently confuses with the target (*money, Monday, muddy, mummy*); a group of cards containing words which are clearly different in pattern and spectral content from the target word (*pig, alligator, ball, television*).

2. Describe the target card to the child; show it to him; allow him to listen to it repeatedly; and then put the target card to the side in a special place. Explain to the child that some of the other cards produce the same word, but some do not. Then shuffle the stimulus cards before the child and place them in a pile.

3. Play the target (*monkey*) card for the child; then immediately play the top card from the stimulus deck. Replace the target card to its special place. The child must now decide whether the stimulus card produces sound that is the *same as* (*yes*) or *different from* (*no*) that on the target card. The child is then requested to place that stimulus card in either a box labeled *yes* or one labeled *no*, whichever he considers appropriate. The child may listen to and compare both target and stimulus cards again if he requests.

4. Repeat this paired listening procedure for subsequent cards in the stimulus deck. Acknowledge correct responses.

5. At a later session, you should ask the child to try making comparable auditory same/different (yes/no) judgments without actually listening to the target card on every trial, but just simply referring to his memory of its acoustic image.

Example C. General purpose: to teach hearing-impaired children to remember sentences in the same order in which they were presented (as in a story, song, poem, or recipe). Hypothetical problem: a severely hearing-impaired child cannot remember and retell a brief story.

1. Before the child arrives, record the sequential material on separate tape-cards and attach an appropriate descriptive picture to each one. Each card may contain one long or two short sentences. Place the cards with attached pictures in sequence, left to right, before the child.

2. Tell the child, for example, "This is a story about a boy and his bicycle." Point to each card/picture in turn and ask the child, "What happened here?" After the child describes the depicted scene in his or her own words (which should resemble those already recorded on the card), play the card to provide the child with a chance to listen to the spoken language associated with that event. Proceed through all of the cards in this way—in sequence.

3. Then place each of the card/pictures on a nearby table, to which you previously have attached a row of numbers. Place each card/picture below its appropriate number in the sequence. Then show the child that the pictures can be detached from the tape-cards and placed beside them. Play each

TABLE 7–2 continued

> tape-card in sequence for the child, associating each one in turn with its appropriate picture.
>
> 4. Ask the child to tell the story in sequence, referring to the pictures if necessary. Play each card for the child as a reward following each correctly recalled item.
> 5. Test the child's ability to identify the sentences acoustically. Demonstrate that you will mix the cards, then mix them, and hand them to the child in random order. The child must listen to each card and place it in its correct position. Then ask the child to repeat the story in sequence. After he or she speaks each numbered sentence, allow the child to listen to the associated card to determine whether he or she was correct. If any errors were made in recall (tape-card placement), he or she should notice them at this time.
> 6. Test the child's ability to identify the sentences acoustically again. This time, however, remove the pictures describing the sequence, leaving only the numbered labels to be associated with the tape-cards. After removing the pictures, mix the cards, and ask the child to listen to each one and place it in its proper position. After he or she places all of the cards, ask for recall of the entire story, letting the child listen to each card after speaking each sentence, as a reward.
> 7. Finally, remove the tape-cards from the table, leaving only the numbered labels. Now ask the child to tell you the story, in sequence, using only the numbers as prompts. Later, you may ask for the complete story without even the numbers as a guide.

auditory discrimination tasks

Discrimination tasks require the child to make same/different decisions about a set of speech stimuli recorded on separate cards or card segments and to indicate his or her response, perhaps by placing the stimulus cards into appropriately labeled containers. For example, a child may both perceive and apply prepositions incorrectly. If you conclude that he or she needs practice hearing the differences between certain prepositions in phrases, you might record ten single-notched cards of the form, "on the table/on the table," and ten cards of the form, "on the table/under the table," or "behind the table." Then, shuffling the twenty cards, you would ask the child to listen to and compare both segments of each card. The child decides whether the spoken items are the same or different, and places the card accordingly into the *SAME* or the *DIFFERENT* box. Of course, the child must already know the *meanings* of the words *same* and *different*. For younger children, you might state the question, "Are these two parts the *same?*", and use boxes labeled *YES* and *NO*. You might also illustrate all of the cards in this set with a picture of a table and/or label each with the phrase, "__ the table." Again, your explanations can be simplified if you make the recordings while the child watches. (see Table 7–2B for a more detailed procedure).

auditory identification tasks

Identification tasks require the child to determine which specific label or which general category describes the acoustic speech stimulus recorded on the tape-card, and to indicate the decision in some way. For example, you may wish to provide extra practice to a particular child in identifying sentences previously used and discussed in class. The sentences may form a small set describing a recent class experience or activity. You may record one of these sentences on each of ten cards and also prepare a set of small tags depicting each of the spoken sentences in some way, either through pictures or print (or both), depending on the age of the child. Attach these to the cards with clips. The sentences might be:

1). "Last week, Melanie had a birthday party."—picture of children at a party.

2). "Melanie's mother baked a cake."—picture of cake.

3). "Mrs. Wells brought enough ice cream for everybody."—picture of children eating ice cream.

First, give the child practice in listening to each tape-card with its identifying label attached. Then remove the labels and place them on the table. Shuffle the set of tape-cards, asking the child to listen to each one in turn. He or she must identify the sentence that was presented by placing the tape-card next to the appropriate picture or printed sentence. In some cases, especially when the number of recorded sentences is small, you might write the complete set of response choices directly on each stimulus card (Figure 7–6). Then you would record each sentence on several tape-cards, shuffle the cards, and ask the child to listen. The child's task is to separate the cards by placing them into boxes that are labeled with the several sentences. Alternatively, you might ask older children to write their identification responses on numbered answer sheets.

General categories of speech patterns may also be used as responses in identification tasks. For example, you may observe that a child does not produce speech with appropriate temporal patterns, judging, therefore, that the child needs practice in recognizing the gross differences between his or her speech and that of normally hearing people. So, you might record a large number of sentences and request the same of the child. Then mix the tape-cards, asking the child to listen to each one, to identify which of the two talkers is speaking, and to respond by sorting the cards into appropriately labeled boxes (*Andrew, Mrs. Dowell*). (See Table 7–2A for more detailed procedure.)

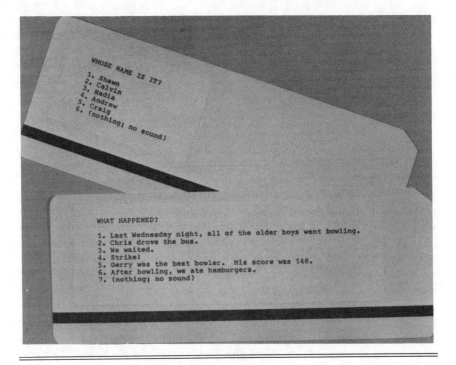

figure 7–6. Examples of audio tape-cards used in identification tasks.

auditory comprehension tasks

Speech *comprehension* tasks require the child to perform activities, write answers to questions, or make complex associations between words, sentences, or sequences—on the basis of questions, information, or instructions recorded on tape-cards. For example, a hearing-impaired child with minimal, although potentially useful, hearing may lack confidence in his or her ability to understand speech through listening alone. Thus, a list of common everyday questions might be recorded on a set of tape-cards (one to a card): 1) "What is your grandfather's name?"; 2) "Where do you eat lunch?"; 3) "What color is your bicycle?"; and 4) "What time is it?" The child is asked to listen to each question in turn and to write the correct answer on an answer sheet or on the card itself.*

---

*Cards can be used repeatedly as response forms, if a sheet of clear plastic laminating film is bonded to the top part of each one. The child writes the response with a special pen, whose marks later can be rubbed off with solvent.

For another child, you might record numerous two-card sets, each containing words that are opposites (for example, north/south, love/hate, and man/woman), and then mix *all* of the cards. The child would be asked to listen to each one and match the associated pairs. In orther cases, you might instruct a child to perform a task (cooking a hamburger, coloring a picture, or assembling a puzzle) on the basis of information given on a series of tape-cards. (See Table 7–2C for a detailed procedure.)

general observations

It should be relatively easy to prepare and evaluate recorded listening materials of the sort described above as a supplement to regular classroom work. There is no limit to the listening tasks that can be created. For most of these applications, you may write the correct response on the back of each tape-card, and you, a student teacher, a teacher-aide, or even another child playing the role of teacher can reward the listener for correct responses. It is important to carefully explain each listening task to the child before he or she begins. It usually is not sufficient merely to hand over a set of cards, some response boxes, and a list of printed instructions. Rather, you must observe the child beginning each new activity to ensure that he or she knows what to do. In general, children who participate in well-planned listening activities quickly learn the assigned tasks and appear to enjoy the independent learning experience. Most teachers tend to assign tape-card tasks to children who have finished other classroom responsibilities and have free time. Also, when a teacher devides the class into small groups for more personal attention, part of the group may be directed to tape-card activities, while the teacher personally works with the remaining children.

Furthermore, it is possible to use tape-card machines as speech training aids with hearing-impaired children by recording your speech models on one track ("instructor") of numerous tape-cards; the messages may be written on cards, if desired. The child listens to each one in turn and attempts to imitate your speech as closely as possible while recording on the other track ("student") (Chapter 9). The child may rerecord his or her speech until satisfied that the two samples match (child's imitation = your model). At a later time, you and the child can discuss similarities and differences in the two recorded sound patterns, comparing personal criteria for judging similarity and difference (that is, the two of you may not agree). For many children, this will be their first experience listening to their own speech without talking (that is, without simultaneously producing voice and moving the articulators). Those who have tried this activity have commented favorably on the opportunity to analyze their own speech patterns without the distraction of concentrating on speech production at the same time.

Occasionally, a child will perform poorly on even carefully planned auditory tape-card tasks. In these cases, it is important to examine the learning situation, to determine why the child experienced unanticipated failure, before proceeding with other listening tasks. One of the following factors may be responsible: 1) your instructions were too complicated for the child's language level; 2) you provided too many response alternatives; 3) the response alternatives were too similar in sound quality; 4) you gave the child too few trials for achievement of an acceptable level of performance; or 5) the listening task was not interesting enough to motivate the child. Once the problem is discovered, you should adapt, by modifying (simplifying) the listening task to place it closer to the child's present range of abilities. Before returning to the original speech materials, you usually will be able to restore the child's self-confidence by presenting another listening task in which he or she previously experienced success.

When a child demonstrates a variety of needs, you must select a particular direction for auditory training. In some instances, this means providing initial listening practice on a level at which the child has been successful, to give him or her confidence in coping with auditory tasks.* Tape-card activities for young hearing-impaired children appear to be most useful for individual *practice*, rather than for independent learning of new language structures or new vocabulary. It is best that the teacher be personally available during those important communication developments.

Usually, a teacher will first sample several of the child's auditory abilities (for example, by administering the GASP!) and then concentrate on tasks in which the child demonstrates moderate success or in which the child seems particularly interested. When the child appears to have difficulty with a particular listening task (such as identification of words), the teacher will confirm that the child can cope with the next lower level (discrimination among the same words) before proceeding.

All things being equal, teachers should apply auditory practice material that interests each individual child, relating, for example, to a recent class activity or to the child's own personal experience. Nevertheless, efficient use of your time, effort, and materials requires that you record audio tape-cards for more general application, so that they can be reused by numerous children with comparable auditory needs; otherwise the time expended in preparing the recordings far exceeds that taken by an individual child to learn

---

*Some children have a great need to develop confidence in their listening skills by showing themselves (and you) that they can use their ears successfully in speech perception tasks. Teachers have reported that previewing a set of tape-cards under conditions of simulated hearing loss (Erber & Zeiser, 1974; Gagné & Erber, 1980; Ross, Duffy, Cooker, & Sargeant, 1973) is very useful in predicting whether a particular set of materials or a special training procedure will be effective with a given hearing-impaired child.

the auditory task. Unfortunately, we have not yet satisfactorily resolved this conflict of objectives.

As a teacher, your philosophy of instruction also will tend to affect the sequence that you use to present stimulus-response tasks. For example, some teachers prefer to develop a child's auditory perception in a stepwise progressive fashion, beginning with low levels of task complexity, such as detection of speech sounds, and then helping the child advance through higher levels as success in listening is demonstrated. Others tend to concentrate on identification or comprehension tasks and assign remedial lower-level activities only when the child demonstrates listening difficulty at the higher levels. Neither method is inherently superior. If you follow each strategy carefully, regardless of the one that you choose, your efforts will lead you to converge* on a set of listening activities that will benefit the child at that specific point in his or her auditory development.

summary

Although many hearing-impaired children develop good listening skills merely from taking part in group conversation, others require carefully monitored individual instruction. Audio tape-card machines can be used effectively to present recorded listening materials for individual practice. Commercially available machines may be supplemented in numerous ways, through attachment of an external microphone, an output amplifier, earphones, and vibrators. This chapter focused on several examples of simple, yet effective, auditory training activities, intended for children with moderate, severe, or profound hearing impairments. These provide practice at the detection, discrimination, identification, and comprehension levels. The recorded materials can be used either for self-instruction by the child or for individual instruction that is closely directed by the teacher or teacher-aide.

---

*Circular reasoning (A Stone Age proverb): "If you intend to construct a wheel that rolls smoothly, it makes little difference which material or shape you start with; used properly and often enough it will become round anyway (although some materials and initial shapes take longer)."

8

use of
the telephone

One of the objectives of any auditory training program is communication through the hearing sense by itself. This is an important goal, in spite of the fact that most daily communication occurs face-to-face and that the hearing-impaired child usually can rely on lipreading cues for auditory-visual communication. The most common instance of communication by listening alone occurs when hearing-impaired children receive speech over the telephone. In recent years, there has been renewed interest in telephone instruction procedures and in special apparatus for use by those with moderate to profound hearing impairments (Castle, 1977, 1978; McLeod & Guenther, 1977).

Communication over the telephone is a central part of the daily lives of most people with normal hearing. It plays a major role in business, family, and personal life. Yet, for many hearing-impaired people who normally communicate through speech, it may be difficult, if not impossible, to use this common device for fluent communication. Some hearing-impaired individuals simply lack experience in listening and thus lack confidence in carrying out the numerous procedures involved in telephone use. Others need special practice to develop appropriate listening and response strategies. Some are unaware of the various accessories and amplification devices that are commercially available to improve communication over the phone. And still others may be using hearing aids that do not adequately couple their telephones acoustically to their ears.

TABLE 8–1. A hearing-impaired listener can receive acoustic messages through the telephone in a variety of ways.

(1) standard telephone handset; no hearing aid.
(2) standard telephone handset; hearing aid used, set to "microphone" (acoustic) input.
(3) standard telephone handset; hearing aid used, set to "telecoil" (electromagnetic) input.
(4) telephone handset with built-in amplifier; no hearing aid.
(5) telephone handset with built-in amplifier; hearing aid used, set to "microphone" (acoustic) input.
(6) telephone handset with built-in amplifier; hearing aid used, set to "telecoil" (electromagnetic) input.

methods of communication

For those hearing-impaired people who use the telephone, there are four main methods of communication (Castle, 1977, 1978): 1) the hearing-impaired person uses a telecommunication device for the deaf (TDD), such as a teleprinter, to convey typed messages over telephone lines to others having similar, compatible equipment; 2) the hearing-impaired person lipreads an oral interpreter (spouse, friend, business associate) who places the call and repeats the other party's messages while the hearing-impaired person responds directly into the phone; 3) the hearing-impaired person speaks directly to the person called but the other party may use only a prearranged, limited set of responses, coded in terms of intensity patterns; and 4) the hearing-impaired person uses speech for both expression and reception. We will be concerned mainly with the latter two methods, which are hearing-oriented procedures.

The hearing-impaired listener may choose from a variety of ways to receive speech acoustically over the telephone (Nielsen & Gilberg, 1978) (Table 8–1). In general, only those with mild hearing losses will use a telephone receiver without a hearing aid (conditions #1 and #4). Some children with moderate to severe hearing losses can cope reasonably well with acoustic coupling to the phone (conditions #2 and #5) and can understand considerable amounts of speech. Many with severe or profound impairments prefer to use their hearing aids on "telecoil" (conditions #3 and #6), because this electromagnetic link provides better speech perception for them.

Individuals differ in their preference for supplementary apparatus even when they have apparently similar hearing abilities. Perhaps this can be attributed to differences in magnetic field strength produced by the telephone handsets of various manufacturers. Or perhaps it is due to subtle differences in hearing aid telecoils, for example, the number of windings or orientation of the coil within the case of the aid. Also, differences in gain or frequency response between the "T" (telephone) or "M" (microphone) setting of a

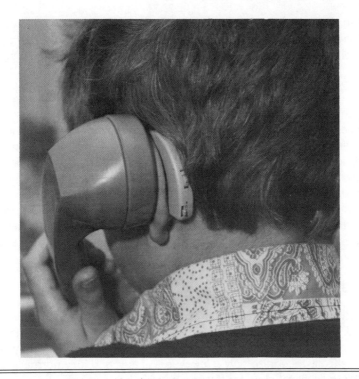

figure 8–1. A hearing-impaired child uses a telephone with a supplementary power amplifier built into the handset. His behind-the-ear hearing aid is set to the "T" (telecoil) position for reception of speech signals radiated electromagnetically from the telephone receiver.

given aid have been reported (Sung, Sung, & Hodgson, 1974). And then, each hearing-impaired child listens to a variety of talkers (parents, friends, and teachers), whose voices probably differ in intensity and quality. Most likely, all of these factors interact in a complicated way with the configuration of hearing sensitivity in the child. To achieve the best speech communication, the child must experiment with each of the conditions listed in Table 8–1 and select one which optimizes intelligibility for him or her (Figure 8–1).

telephone communication ability

Most hearing-impaired children can be subdivided into one of three general levels of telephone communication ability:

Group 1

Children who communicate fluently over the telephone (without visual contact) with few errors and little need for repetition by the talker. These

children typically score between 8 to 10 on the GASP! sentence comprehension subtest (Chapter 4). They also respond equally well on other auditory
comprehension tasks when these are administered with the mouth covered.

Group 2

Children who can communicate successfully when the talker has the
patience to repeat frequently, and knows their auditory vocabulary and language limitations. These children may be able to identify numerous words
in isolation, but they tend to have difficulty with connected speech presented
at a normal rate. They may score from 0 to about 7 on the GASP! auditory
comprehension subtest. Some have very little confidence in their auditory
abilities, especially when the talker's mouth is not visible. Therefore, in many
instances, their auditory test performance is not indicative of their capability.
With guided practice in listening over the telephone, they may learn and gain
confidence rapidly.

Group 3

Children for whom special acoustic intensity-pattern codes must be
devised. These are children whose auditory abilities are so poor that they
receive only the basic intensity patterns of speech reliably. They may be able
to acoustically recognize only a few words, if any, and they normally require
simultaneous visual cues for fluent comprehension of speech.

A simple guide to evaluating a child's telephone communication skills
is presented in Table 8–2. Such an evaluation requires an informal judgment
by the teacher or hearing specialist, who observes the child's use of the
telephone under various conditions.

One direct method of evaluation is through a simulated telephone
conversation, placing the child by a telephone and asking an assistant to
ring while you the teacher observe the child's communication behavior. The
assistant may ask the child ordinary questions about family, friends, pets,
recent vacation trip, or sports, while you watch and listen. Observe how the
child begins and ends the conversation and how easily he or she communicates. Note, also, his or her ability to understand by listening alone, to ask
clarifying questions, whether he or she takes turns and avoids long silences,
how the child makes him- or herself understood, and the level of self-confidence. The same observations may be made while conversing with the child
yourself, when the child does not have a hearing person nearby to provide
suggestions or help. Also, specifically evaluate the child's ability to use the
telephone to acquire information. For example, ask to be phoned while
pretending that you represent a movie theater, department store, museum,
or zoo; or suggest that the child actually phone one of those places to obtain
information.

TABLE 8–2. A simple guide that can be used to evaluate a child's telephone communication skills.

I. Brief questionnaire
   1. Do you want to use the telephone? Why?
      a. Personal, social (friends, relatives)
      b. Obtain information (shops, organizations)
      c. Business (coworkers, customers)
   2. Is there a microphone/telephone (M/T) switch on your hearing aid? How do you use it?
      Does the M/T switch work properly?
      Does the internal induction coil work properly?
   3. Do you already use a telephone? yes/no
      How?
      a. TDD (teletypewriter)
      b. Voice code ("no/yes-yes/please repeat")
      c. Oral interpreter (friend, relative, business associate)
      d. Speech communication (both talk and listen)
   4. How often do you use a telephone? _____times per day/week
      a. Whom do you talk to? Why?
      b. Do you ever telephone other people? Who? Why?
   5. What sort of telephone do you have at home?
      a. Telephone amplifier/no telephone amplifier
      b. Bell/gliding tone
      c. Does your telephone (and accessories) work properly?
   6. Who answers the telephone at home? Do *you* answer the telephone when no one else is at home?
   7. Do you understand speech over the telephone?
      a. Are some people easier to understand than others? Why?
      b. What do you do when you don't understand someone's speech?
   8. Do other people understand *your* speech over the telephone?
      a. Do certain people understand you better than others? Why?
      b. What do you do when someone doesn't understand your speech?
II. Best listening conditions (determined by test/judgment)
   1. Preferred ear for listening: left/right
   2. Telephone amplifier/no telephone amplifier
   3. Hearing aid switch position: M/T
   4. Use of supplementary induction coil in (or on) telephone receiver: yes/no
   5. Use of noise-isolating rubber cuff on telephone receiver: yes/no
III. Basic skills
   1. Holding the telephone receiver in the proper position with regard to hearing aid, ear, and mouth
   2. Recognition of common telephone sounds
      a. Incoming call: ringer bell/gliding tone
         i. in same room
        ii. from adjacent room
       iii. from outside house

TABLE 8–2. continued

---

      b. Dialed call: other person's phone ringing
      c. Engaged (busy) signal
      d. Poor connection
      e. Number disconnected (recording)
      f. Wrong number (live person)
   3. Dialing
      a. Standard procedure
         i. Own phone
         ii. Public phone
         iii. Business phone (first obtain outside line)
      b. Long distance
         i. Via telephone operator
           —to dialed number
           —to specific person
         ii. Direct dialed
      c. "Collect" calls (charge to other person)
      d. Emergency calls (to police station, fire department, ambulance)
      e. Calls to telephone company business office (to report own telephone out of order)
   4. Organizational skills
      a. Find number in telephone directory
         i. White pages (alphabetized by name)
         ii. Yellow pages (alphabetized by subject)
      b. Maintain personal telephone directory (frequently used numbers)
      c. Telephone bills
         i. Installation cost
         ii. Rental expenses
         iii. Monthly charges
IV. Speech-perception ability
   1. Speech-sound detection
   2. Speech-sound identification
   3. Word/phrase identification
   4. Sentence (question/statement) comprehension
   5. Voice (talker) identification
V. Speech-production ability
   1. Speech-sound identification
   2. Word/phrase identification
   3. Sentence (question/statement) comprehension
VI. Need for visible cues
   1. Talker in same room
      a. Mouth/face visible
      b. Mouth/face covered
   2. Talker in adjacent (or nearby) room, talker accessible
   3. Talker in separate building (remote location); talker inaccessible
VII. Need for cooperation during conversation
   1. Experienced hearing therapist

TABLE 8-2. continued

> 2. Familiar person (friend, relative)
> 3. Volunteer listener (helpful, but inexperienced)
> 4. Unfamiliar person who does not expect call (shop owner)
> 5. Business or organization that does not expect call (theater)
> VIII. Conversational skills
> 1. Initiate conversation
> 2. Obtain/provide information; ask questions
> 3. Take turns; avoid silences
> 4. Use telephone strategies when necessary
>   a. Give instructions to talker (request repetition, louder/softer/slower speech)
>   b. Repeat; guess; take chances in communication
>   c. Confirm message reception ("Did you say...?")
> 5. Write important information; take message for another person
> 6. End conversation

use of closed-circuit telephone systems

Initial telephone evaluation and training can be greatly enhanced through the use of a special closed-circuit telephone system provided by the telephone company (usually free of charge).* These systems typically consist of two standard dial (or push-button) telephone units with handsets, connected by long cables to a central power supply, amplifier, and ringing terminal. In addition, each handset may contain a supplementary amplifier, assembled by the telephone company.

This type of system has been used in three different configurations: 1) The teacher and child sit within the same room (at a 2 to 4 meter distance from one another). Each holds a telephone handset and communicates acoustically over the telephone line. The teacher's mouth is covered by a large piece of cardboard, but this barrier may be lowered to provide visible cues for speech when the child needs clarification or help. This introductory near condition is intended to familiarize the child with basic telephone procedures. 2) The teacher and child sit in adjacent rooms, each out of sight of the other, but the teacher still is accessible for help when the child requires it (Figure 8-2). This intermediate condition helps the child develop a greater amount of independence and confidence during telephone communication, because most of the time no one else is in the room. The child is motivated to carry on the conversation independently, if possible. 3) The teacher and the child are in rooms remote from one another (a very long telephone

---

*For example, the Teletrainer, distributed by the Bell Telephone Company.

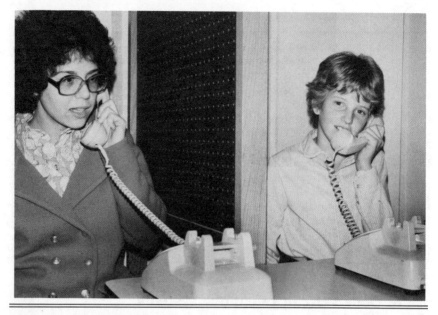

figure 8–2. A teacher helps a hearing-impaired child practice speech communication over the telephone. The teacher sits in an adjacent room, to provide auditory-
visual assistance if the child requires it.

extension cable may be purchased or assembled for this purpose). They
may be on different floors of the same building or even in nearby buildings.
This remote condition closely simulates a real conversational situation and
forces the child to be self-reliant in developing the conversation, acquiring
information, and requesting clarification strategies when necessary. The teacher
is not accessible; the child must solve any communication problems alone.

These three degrees of teacher accessibility represent a progression
from a setting of closely supervised communication to one of independent
communication. Not all children can progress through all three levels. Some
lack the maturity of self-confidence required; some lack the hearing capacity
to communicate fluently without visible speech cues. The teacher's role is
to help each child achieve his or her auditory communication potential in
accordance with hearing capacity.

"tracking" and telephone communication practice

The special evaluation and practice procedure known as "tracking" (De-
Filippo & Scott, 1978) has been applied to telephone communication. Originally developed to evaluate lipreading efficiency, this same basic method
can be used with minor modifications, both for general auditory training

(Chapter 5), and to provide practice at the identification level to hearing-impaired children listening over the telephone.

With this method, you would read portions of a prepared story or article over a telephone system. The child listens through a telephone handset and attempts to repeat word-for-word what you say. You present the material in small segments, whose lengths (whole sentences, phrases, words, or even phonemes) depend upon the ease with which the child seems to be receiving speech at that particular time. Although, *you* would choose most of the remedial auditory communication strategies when difficulty occurs, the *child* also may suggest methods of clarification. Thus, it may be necessary for you to repeat, exaggerate, increase your voice level, change syntax, provide synonyms for words, and so forth (Erber, 1979c; Erber & Greer, 1973).

The following arbitrary rule is used to avoid excessive telephone communication delays when the child cannot understand a message segment—if he or she is unable to identify a word or phrase after three repetitions, and also after application of three different acoustic strategies, then that message segment is simply bypassed; however, you should make note of the difficult item for later discussion with the child (see Table 8–3 for examples of some words and phrases that were difficult for one particular hearing-impaired listener to identify over the telephone).

The total number of words in the story or article is divided by the total time (in minutes) required to complete the repetition task. The result is the "tracking rate," expressed in words per minute.

A typical practice session may consist of: 1) 10 minutes of informal (auditory-visual) discussion of previously successful acoustic strategies (for example, use of synonyms or rephrasing of entire sentences) and a brief orientation to the content of the day's story, including an introduction to proper nouns (names, places) in the text that will be used; 2) 20 to 30 minutes of auditory "tracking" via a telephone system and personal hearing aids, or occasionally through the child's amplification system alone, bypassing the telephone; and 3) 10 minutes of (auditory-visual) review of auditory difficulties encountered on that day, including examination of unfamiliar words and phrases, especially those that were difficult or impossible to communicate. The goal is to help the child understand his or her capabilities and persistent difficulties (perhaps, the inability to distinguish / m, n / or / v, z /). In addition, the relative value of various remedial strategies are discussed with the child (Table 8–4).

The results of several tracking practice sessions are shown in Figure 8–3. The participants in the work were two severely hearing-impaired 18-year-old males. Both were regular hearing aid users, and expressed a strong desire to improve their auditory communication over the telephone. These listeners already could easily identify telephone signals (dial tone, busy signal), and could engage in simple conversations with family members and close friends with normal hearing. They merely needed practice in listening and

TABLE 8–3. Auditory identification errors demonstrated by an 18-year-old severely hearing-impaired listener, while using the "Tracking" procedure to practice speech communication over the telephone. Many of these auditory errors can be explained simply on the basis of vowel or consonant confusions.

Talker's Spoken Stimulus	Listener's Incorrect Identification
big	good
back	fast
ten	six
soon	same
pain	team
win	limp
rolled	would
end	hear
fooled	told, sold
jet	trip, kid
me	knee
death	desk
faced	stayed
get even	next season
kind	time
fareway	area
talented	challenged
learned	won
late	night
even more	easy four
kicker	fielder
made	need
half	pass
winning	women

development of special strategies. As can be seen, both listeners improved their auditory tracking rate (words per minute) while communicating with a normally hearing clinician. However, their telephone performance after 6 to 7 sessions still was considerably below the rate that they could achieve through auditory-visual communication (face-to-face) while using their personal hearing aids.

Some strategies that have been suggested to clarify telephone communication are listed in Table 8–4a&b (Castle, 1977). All are occasionally helpful. For example, you may spell out words letter-by-letter; however, this approach can introduce problems of its own if the child misunderstands the letter names themselves. For example, frequent confusions occur between the letters f, t, p and also between f, s, x. You can try placing a difficult word into a more familiar context (for example, rolled: "The two boys rolled down

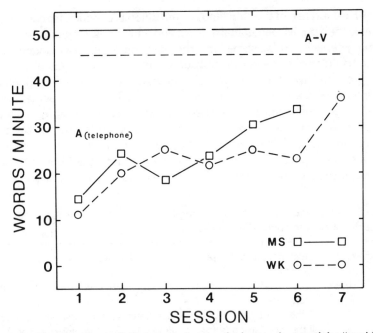

figure 8–3. Results of seven listening sessions in which a teacher used the "tracking" (repetition) procedure to provide practice in speech perception over the telephone to two severely hearing-impaired teenagers. The material consisted of brief stories about sports heroes. Their auditory-visual repetition rates (words/ minute) also are shown for comparison.

the hill in a red wagon."). This strategy is useful, but it can fail if the child is unable to understand even the clarifying context by hearing alone. And using code words to cue letters (Table 8–5) can be tedious since not all code words are equally familiar or intelligible to all children. You probably will need to construct a different set for each child according to individual vocabulary and auditory capabilities. Of all the clarifying strategies tried, perhaps the most effective requires the child to guide the talker to modify his or her own speech according to a judged deficiency. In other words, the child may instruct the talker to increase his or her voice level, repeat a phrase, say the last two words more slowly, and so forth.

Most children, in addition to learning a repertoire of specific communication strategies, have learned to sustain their auditory attention over long periods of time during telephone practice without getting frustrated. They have learned how to ask carefully worded clarifying questions—rather than simply asking, "What did you say?", they may ask, "Are you still talking about your new dress?" Each child who has participated in this work also has gained considerable confidence in his or her auditory abilities, and especially in the ability to manage a telephone conversation.

Through use of the "tracking" or repetition procedure, teachers directly observe their pupils' perceptual abilities and limitations, language facility, and learning capacity. At the same time, they develop a subjective understanding of the usefulness of particular oral/aural communication strategies.

For effective "tracking" to be carried out, several weeks of orientation are beneficial both for the child and for the teacher. Before actual practice begins, agreement must be reached on special code words for letters and special code phrases for cueing certain strategies (for example, "say again" to indicate that a difficult word will be repeated, or "different sentence" to indicate that a particular phrase will be used in a different context). And of course, if the hearing-impaired child's *speech* is only marginally intelligible

TABLE 8—4a. Some ways that a hearing-impaired child may request help during a telephone conversation (Castle, 1977).

REPEAT: Repeat that please. Repeat the whole thing. Repeat the (*first, second, last*) word.

REPHRASE: Say it a different way please. Say another word that means the same thing.

SPELL: Spell the word please. What is the (*first, second, last*) sound/letter? Spell the word in code (use code words). Say the alphabet until you come to the right letter.

WHICH NUMBER?: Say each number, one at a time. Count numbers until you come to the right number.

WHAT TOPIC?: Did you say _____? Are you talking about _____? Are you still talking about _____? What is the most important word in the sentence? What are you talking about?

PROVIDE CHOICES: Examples: Should I come today or tomorrow? I want you to pick me up at 4:30. O.K.?

CLARIFY/VERIFY: I don't understand your speech. Talk louder/softer. Talk slower. Talk normally.

TABLE 8—4b. Some ways that a teacher may guide a child's speech communication during a telephone conversation.

CLARIFY/VERIFY: That's right (O.K.)! No, that's wrong! I don't understand your speech. Talk louder/softer. Talk slower. What do you want me to do? Please repeat.

PROVIDE

DIRECTION: Let's talk about something different. I'm talking about something new. I'm talking about _____. I'm still talking about _____.

SPECIFY STRATEGY: I'm going to start over. I'm going to say the (*first, second, last*) word again. I'm going to say that again a different way. This is the (*first, second, last*) sound/letter: _____. I will spell the word (in code). I will count the numbers.

TABLE 8–5. Some multisyllabic code words that were used to cue letters during telephone communication practice with two severely hearing-impaired children.

Child 1:	Child 2:
a —anteater	a —alphabet
b —bad baby	b —bacteria
c —cocoanut	c —constitution
d —Doctor Doolittle	d —dandelion
e —encyclopedia	e —elephant
f —football	f —Florida
g —girl friend	g —gorilla
h —hot dog	h —helicopter
i —ice cream	i —ice cube
j —jelly beans	j —jingle bells
k —kangaroo	k —Kansas City
l —lighthouse	l —lollipop
m—microphone	m—milkman
n —New South Wales	n —New York
o —octopus	0 —Oklahoma
p —Prince Charles	p —potato
q —Queen Elizabeth	q —quarter
r —Round Table	r —Rhode Island
s —Saturday	s —slimy snake
t —television	t —toothbrush
u —United States	u —underdog
v —vegetable	v —violin
w —weekend	w —watermelon
x —extra special	x —Xanadu
y —yellow bird	y —yesterday
z —zebra stripes	z —zoo animals

to the teacher over the telephone (without visible cues), then auditory communication is likely to break down repeatedly unless the child recognizes the need to exert effort to make him- or herself understood acoustically .

practice with prerecorded messages

A significant number of severely hearing-impaired students want to communicate over the telephone for social and practical purposes, yet many express great anxiety about receiving information from a live talker whom they do not know and whom they cannot see to lipread. However, most of them exhibit little fear of listening to speech that has been recorded, as over a tape-card playback system, a phonograph, or a tape recorder. And many are quite capable of understanding speech acoustically, scoring between 6 and 10 on the sentence comprehension subtest of the GASP!

Given this dilemma, numerous hearing-impaired children have been practicing listening to *prerecorded* messages over the telephone. The purpose is to give them extensive listening experiences without requiring direct verbal interaction. Later, after the children feel more comfortable about using a telephone for actual auditory communication, they are introduced to interactive conversation.

At first, children are asked simply to dial and listen to prerecorded messages about the current time, weather, theater schedules, and so forth (Table 8–6). They use a standard telephone with a handset amplifier in combination with their personal hearing aids. This activity has been reasonably successful, but children often complain that some of the recorded talkers present their information at too rapid a rate and with insufficient clarity. In some cases, the recordings themselves are of poor quality; electrical background noise and/or static makes listening difficult. Numerous recorded messages have since been rated from high to low in intelligibility and are selected accordingly for listening practice.

More recently, the commercial messages have been supplemented with specially recorded closed-loop cassettes played through a Bell Telephone Teletrainer, the recordings so contrived that they contain content and structure modeled after those of actual prerecorded telephone messages available to the public. Most of these, however, have been greatly simplified with regard to their vocabulary and language (Table 8–7a). The taped talker articulates slowly and carefully as he or she presents each message. Each presentation

TABLE 8–6. Example of typical commercial recorded message, along with information relevant to a teacher who wishes to use the dialed recording to provide listening practice for a hearing-impaired child.

Tivoli Theatre (725-0220): male voice, low pitch; recorded in reverberant room, low-frequency emphasis; moderate amount of tape hiss; recorded message does not repeat (redialing necessary).

"Thank you for calling the Tivoli Theatre, located at 6350 Delmar, two blocks west of Skinker in the University City Loop. Our program for Friday, February 20th includes two rock-and-roll films. At 7:15, it's *Pink Floyd* in concert, and at 9:00 o'clock the Ramones return in the classic, *Rock and Roll High School.* Our program for Saturday, February 21st: two Woody Allen (2-second gap in tape) ... *Sleeper* at 3:45 and 7:15, and *Love and Death* at 5:30 and 9:00 o'clock. Tickets are three-fifty for adults, three dollars for students with an ID and senior citizens, and two dollars for children. For further information, or business calls, please dial 725-0221, after 6:00 o'clock. Thanks again for calling the Tivoli, and have a nice day."

(Total time = 49 seconds)

lasts about 30 seconds and repeats continuously. Other recorded messages have also been constructed containing useful information such as the daily lunch menu and after-school activities (Table 8–7b).

A printed set of questions guides each child's listening and establishes a purpose for the activity ("What's for lunch today?"). A fill-in-the-blank format also has been used, in which parts of the actual spoken sentence are given, and the child is asked to supply the remainder. To make initial listening easier, three or four possible alternate responses may be listed. Later, as the child's confidence increases, the printed alternatives are withdrawn and the task presented in open-set format.

The use of these carefully recorded messages has reduced students' anxiety about telephone use. The talker's speech rate can gradually be increased, before resuming listening practice with actual prerecorded messages available to the general public.

use of a question-answer format for practice

Another proven practice technique requires the teacher to ask questions of the hearing-impaired child over the telephone. This task provides practice at the comprehension level.

TABLE 8–7a. Samples of prerecorded messages used for telephone practice: Community Activities.

1. Weather information:
   Thank you for calling the Weatherline. The temperature today will reach _____(17°c, 25°c, 31°c). It will be partly cloudy and _____(cooler, windy, warmer). The weather for Saturday probably will be _____ (warmer, sunny, rainy).
         What weather is predicted for Saturday?

2. The Zoo:
   Thank you for calling the Zoo. The zoo is open from _____(7 A.M. to 12 noon, 9 A.M. to 5 P.M., 9 A.M. to 8 P.M.). There is a special lecture on _____ (birds, elephants, monkeys) this Friday at _____(10 A.M., 1:30 P.M., 4 P.M.). The admission price is _____($1.50, 1.00, 2.00) for adults and _____ (75¢, 50¢, $1.00) for children under _____(8, 11, 13).
     How much does it cost for an 10-year-old child to get into the zoo?

3. Art Museum:
   You will find the Art Museum on _____(Alexander, Pine, Victoria) Street. It is open every day except _____(Sunday, Saturday, Wednesday) from _____(9 to 9, 11 to 4, 10 to 2). This month, our special exhibit is a collection of drawings by _____(Pablo Picasso, Leonardo da Vinci, Michelangelo.)
         When is the art museum closed?

TABLE 8–7b. Samples of prerecorded messages used for telephone practice: School-Related Activities.

1. Lunch Menu:
   The lunch menu for Friday will include: broiled _____(fish, chicken, pork chops). The vegetable will be _____(salad, peas, green beans). We also will have rolls and bread. _____(Ice cream, Cake, Bananas) will be served for dessert.

         What will be served for dessert on Friday?

2. After School:
   Thursday after school, we will show the movie, _____(The Wizard of Oz, The Sound of Music, Peter Pan), in _____(the music room, Classroom #7, the conference room). Also, we will have a _____ (jewelry-making, karate, cake-decorating) demonstration in _____ (the main lobby, the dining room, Classroom #2).

         Where should you go to see the movie on Thursday?

3. The Circus:
   This Saturday, _____(the older boys, the younger boys, all of the girls) will go_____ (on a bus, in a car, on a train) to see the circus. It will cost ($1.50, 2.00, 3.25) for each person. We will leave at _____(9:30 A.M., 10:00 A.M., 1:00P.M.).

         Who is going to see the circus?

A large number of simple questions with one-word answers have been constructed (similar to Harvard Psycho-Acoustic Laboratory Test #12, of the 1940s). The questions refer to body parts, colors, numbers, days, arithmetic, and so on (Table 8–8). The questions vary in length from 5 to 15 syllables. These are questions that most hearing-impaired children of age 10 years and older can answer easily when presented in print.

After introductory face-to-face practice, the teacher and child take their places at each end of a telephone system (either closed-circuit or connected through a switchboard). The child is instructed to answer each question as

TABLE 8–8. Examples of questions asked by teachers during telephone practice.

What color is the sky?
What number comes between six and eight?
What grows on top of your head?
How many eyes do you have?
What day comes after Tuesday?
What do you use to sweep a floor?
Who puts out fires in buildings?
What shape is a ball?
What time do you eat lunch?
What is the opposite of soft?

TABLE 8–9. Questions answered in 30 minutes by 10 severely hearing-impaired children, age range 12 to 15 years. Data from three 10-minute sessions are pooled. Two methods of scoring were used: (a) number of questions answered correctly; (b) percentage of questions answered correctly (number answered divided by number attempted). Both auditory (telephone alone) and auditory-visual scores (telephone plus TV image of the talker's face) are shown for each child.

	Auditory alone			Auditory-visual (A-V)		
Listener	#Att.	#Comp.	%	#Att.	#Comp.	%
R.A.A.G.	45	21	46.7	203	199	98.0
J.A.H	43	20	46.5	137	127	92.7
J.T.J	40	15	37.5	96	89	92.7
M.E.S.	49	18	36.7	196	194	99.0
M.C.S.	43	15	34.9	174	164	94.2
C.R.F.	48	15	31.3	240	238	99.2
R.A.G.	35	7	20.0	182	176	96.7
C.M.A.	32	5	15.6	97	93	95.9
J.H.J.	42	3	7.1	158	152	96.2
M.A.Y.	33	1	3.0	179	173	96.6

Note: #att. = number attempted; #comp. = number comprehended, that is, correctly answered.

quickly as possible. If unable to understand the question, the child is told to repeat that part of the question that he or she *can* identify. The child may request a repetition or clarification of the part he or she *cannot* identify, or the entire question if necessary. If after two (complete or partial) repetitions, the child still is unable to identify any part of the question correctly, the teacher selects from among several strategies. For example, you may present only the key words in the question separately for identification of topic. You may again present the entire question, word by word, with the child repeating after each word. Or you may present verbal prompts, in an attempt to convey the general content of the question (for example, "What time do you eat lunch?" ... "Look at the clock."). The amount of time required to attempt each strategy will vary for different questions, children, and teachers. Your decision to continue with a question, or to bypass it and proceed instead to the next question, will depend on the child's interest and attentiveness, his or her motivation to achieve a high level of comprehension, and your reaction to communication difficulty.

A child's performance may be expressed in at least two ways: 1) the number of questions answered correctly in a period of time (9 questions in 10 minutes); or 2) the percentage of questions answered correctly in a period of time (9 questions answered out of 12 attempted, or 75 percent, in 10 minutes). Scores obtained for a group of ten 12- to 15-year-old severely hearing-impaired children are shown in Table 8–9. Although their auditory-

TABLE 8–10. Examples of questions asked by hearing-impaired children to practice speech communication over the telephone.

To a secretary in the school office:
What is your job?
What things do you do in your job?
How long have you worked here?
What did you do before you started working here?
What do you like about your job? What do you not like?
Do you have any children? How old are they? What are their names? Where do they go to school?
Where are you going during the holidays?

To a student teacher:
Where were you born? What did you like to do when you were a teenager?
Where do you live? Where did you go to college? What are your favorite subjects?
When is your birthday? What is your favorite color? . . . favorite football (baseball, soccer, hockey) team?
What sort of food do you like to cook (eat)?
What are your hobbies? What will you do this weekend?
What kind of movies do you like to see? Tell me some movies that you have seen.

To a teacher:
What pages should I read in the science book?
When are we having a test?
Where are we going tomorrow on our field trip? How much money should I bring? What time are we leaving from school?
Which questions should I answer from the social studies book?
When does the bus leave for the basketball game tonight?
What kind of dog do you have? Did it have puppies yet? How many?
Did you fix your car? What was wrong with it? How much did it cost? It's so expensive; why do you keep it?

---

visual scores (percentage comprehension) are similar, large differences in *auditory* performance among the children are apparent, presumably resulting from differences in auditory capacity and also listening experience.

At other times, the procedure has been reversed somewhat, and the hearing-impaired child is required to obtain answers to questions. Here, the task need not be so formal; it is not necessary to time practice sessions or keep score, although you may. Give the child the name of someone on the school staff, his or her telephone (extension) number, and a set of suggested questions as the basis for a brief telephone "conversation". The child's task is to obtain answers to these questions and perhaps even to extend the dialogue (Table 8–10). The selected staff member receives a minimal amount of practice regarding strategies that a child is likely to use (Table 8–4a), and also is shown ways that he or she can help guide the conversation (Table 8–4b). This sort of listening activity is recommended for those children who seem to have the required auditory abilities and also the confidence necessary to engage in extended conversaton with a live talker.

intensity-pattern codes

Most children with profound hearing impairments must use special intensity-pattern codes for speech communication over the telephone. With this method, the hearing-impaired child essentially controls the direction and structure of the conversation.

In one approach, the child words successive messages as yes/no questions, and the normally hearing speaker at the other end of the telephone line answers in one of three ways: "NO" (one syllable); "O.K.," "that's right,"

TABLE 8–11. Example of a "message table" for transmitting complex messages over the telephone through use of an elaborate intensity-pattern code (from McLeod & Guenther, 1977).

ROW: This number is counted out *first.*		COLUMN: This number is counted out *second.*				
		1	2	3	4	5
	1	Can I speak with someone else?	What have you been doing?	What are you doing today?	What are you doing tonight?	How was your weekend?
	2	Will you have lunch with me?	Can we go out?	Can you visit me?	Can I visit you?	When will you get there/here?
	3	Will you have dinner with me?	Suggest an earlier time.	Suggest a later time.	Have a nice day.	When are you leaving?
	4	Do you want to go out to eat?	I cannot keep our date.	I need your help. Come over.	I don't understand.	Count out the time.
	5	I understand.	I miss you.	Your place.	My business place.	My home/ apartment/ room.

or "yes-yes" (two syllables); or "Please repeat" or "I don't understand" (three or more syllables). These reasonably distinct speech signals may be sent by speaking or by tapping or blowing comparable beat patterns into the telephone mouthpiece (Castle, 1977). Most profoundly hearing-impaired children can easily distinguish among the three patterns. Obviously, this method limits the nature and scope of the telephone conversations that can be held. Still, many children find it very useful for communicating with hearing people who know the code. For example, a hearing-impaired child may use this method to call his or her parents from a friend's house and ask for a ride home at a particular time ("Can you pick me up at John's house at 4:00?").

A more elaborate communication scheme involving an intensity-pattern code has been devised by McLeod and Guenther (1977). When applying this procedure, both communicators may count out a prearranged number sequence that denotes a particular message—greetings, caller's name, instructions, and responses (see Table 8–11). The hearing-impaired communicator also may use connected speech to convey messages not included in the set. This method allows considerably more flexibility in telephone conversation than does the basic one described above, but it requires more careful preparation, attention, persistence, and experience with special speech communication methods by both the hearing and the hearing-impaired communicator. Moreover, profoundly hearing-impaired children typically require considerable practice with either method before they can transmit or receive meaningful messages over the telephone.

summary

Hearing-impaired children exhibit different degrees of ability to communicate by speech over the telephone. Their conversational fluency will depend on hearing loss, general linguistic knowledge, adequacy of the acoustic link between the telephone, hearing aid, and ear, experience in receiving messages without visible cues, application of clarification strategies, their own acoustic speech intelligibility, and the patience and assistance of the hearing people with whom they communicate. Your role as teacher or hearing specialist is to eliminate as many of these barriers as possible and help each child maximize his or her potential for telephone communication. You may accomplish these goals by employing a progressive approach to communication independence, in which you gradually decrease your accessibility to the hearing-impaired child. Numerous special listening activities may be applied for practice as well: attention to details in recorded messages; repetition of connected discourse ("tracking"); participation in simulated conversations (such as question-answer tasks); and application of special codes devised especially for use over the telephone.

9

speech
development

This chapter describes a method of speech development and instruction that is based on *acoustic* stimulation of the impaired ear. In this approach, most of the instructor's speech models are presented with the mouth covered, or at least out of the pupil's field of vision. The child compares the perceptual qualities of his or her own speech with those of the model while attempting to imitate it.

acoustic methods of speech instruction

Recently, a long-term observation study of the acoustic method was completed by Edson (1978), who attempted to develop self-correction of speech in four severely hearing-impaired children age 10 to 15 years. She found that while all of the children were able to learn to accurately imitate her acoustic speech (and language) models, they did not maintain the same precision of production during daily conversation. Edson concluded that these older students had become too dependent on vision and kinesthesia (internally feeling the positions, pressures, and movements of their own articulators) to convert to acoustic cues for speech monitoring and control. She also reasoned that it would be difficult to achieve success in acoustic speech instruction in an educational environment that does not strongly stress audition (to the exclusion of vision) during other communication-oriented activities. Similar views have been expressed by other active practitioners of the method (Asp, 1973; Beebe, 1953; Ling, 1976; Pollack, 1970). Nevertheless, this project and other recent classroom experiences have demonstrated that acoustic speech correction is a potentially effective method for use with many hearing-impaired children, assuming that the method is introduced early and applied consistently.

If a child learns to use only vision and kinesthesia for speech feedback, accurate speech production may be limited to only those articulations which the child can see or feel clearly. In addition, it is impractical for a child to constantly evaluate his or her speech by self-observation in a mirror or by reference to the instructor's facial or gestural cues. In recent years, researchers have developed numerous electronic devices to help hearing-impaired children monitor and control various components of their speech through external tactile and visual feedback (Boothroyd & Decker, 1973; Nickerson, Kalikow, & Stevens, 1976; Willemain & Lee, 1971). Unfortunately, there has been limited success in carryover outside the speech laboratory, where the special feedback apparatus is not present.

More importantly, nonacoustic methods of speech instruction have a far-reaching effect, beyond intelligibility. The child who perceives only the visible aspects of the speech of others is likely to develop a *visual code* for receptive language. This same child probably monitors his or her own speech *tactually and/or kinesthetically*. It is not at all clear how the child would establish an organizational, or linguistic, framework for speech communication, whether in terms of optical or kinesthetic symbols. It is speculated that, for *speech reception*, a child might transform observed oral articulations into a sequence of idealized mouth-images, and would repeatedly refer to this remembered pattern to decode (lipread) what was said (DeFilippo, 1980). For speech *production*, he or she might try to reproduce a sequence of the same idealized mouth-images—forming words so as to be lipread by others (Conrad, 1972; Jenson, 1971; Ling, 1976). In either case, it is likely that only surface (visible) articulation plays a prominent role in the reception or production of speech.

In contrast, people with normal hearing communicate mainly through the *sounds* of speech, and the visible position and movement cues are merely byproducts of that sound production. If the hearing-impaired child were to practice using hearing (or even vibrotactile perception) for communication, he or she might acquire some form of acoustic code for both recognizing and producing spoken language. The result would be more successful interaction with hearing people, for whom acoustic coding is customary. Further, the child would have a useful feedback mechanism available at all times—hearing aids, delivering sound through his or her (impaired) ears.

What follows is a brief review of current knowledge about the typical speech production behavior of numerous hearing-impaired children, and then an exploration of ways in which a teacher can use a particular child's (impaired) hearing to develop his or her speech acoustically.

common speech and language errors

Many children exhibit speech errors that seem to be a function of their impaired perception (Gold, 1980; Smith, 1975). Often, the sounds that a child omits or misarticulates are those that he or she does not detect or perceive clearly, either through audition or lipreading.

intensity patterns

Errors are likely to occur in rhythm, stress pattern, syllable rate, or overall duration of a sentence (Hudgins & Numbers, 1942). These aspects of an utterance are characterized by intensity changes in speech, somewhat independent of pitch, articulation, and the message content. Typically, hearing-impaired children utter syllables in speech too slowly, do not adequately differentiate in production between stressed and unstressed syllables, improperly insert or fill pauses in running speech (even producing a syllable with no voice), and often group syllables inappropriately, distorting the rhythm of the utterance (Figure 9–1). It is claimed that some of these disturbances in the acoustic pattern result from inadequate breath control during each speech production (Nickerson, 1975).

voice pitch and quality

Voice pitch errors tend to fall into two main categories: the child may exhibit an inappropriate average pitch, and/or may change pitch improperly. Many children produce a voice pitch that is abnormally high. Monotone voice and abrupt pitch breaks also are common problems. The intonation contour of a sentence may not be appropriate to its content (for example, a lack of pitch change in the sentence, "Do you want a red pen or a blue pen?"). Many of these voice pitch errors are thought to be the result of improper muscle use or control (Martony, 1968; Nickerson, 1975).

The voice quality of hearing-impaired children has often been described as "breathy" or "tense" (Calvert, 1962). This has been attributed to inappropriate positioning of the vocal folds during speech.

articulation

Poor control of the raising or lowering of the velum (soft palate) is a source of difficulty in the speech of many hearing-impaired children. Inappropriate velar control can contribute to confusion for the listener attempting to distinguish voiced stops / b, d, g / from their nasal counterparts / m, n, ŋ /. Often it is difficult for the hearing-impaired child to produce intelligible consonant clusters containing nasals, such as / nt, nd, mp /.

Inability to produce appropriate vowel qualities also is a problem common to many hearing-impaired children. The child may produce a sound

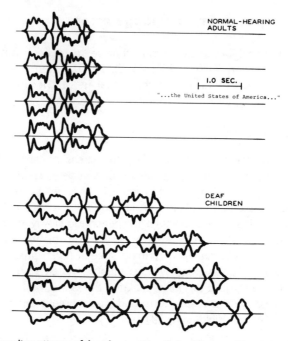

figure 9–1. Intensity patterns of the phrase, "the United States of America," as spoken by four teachers with normal hearing (top) and by four children with profound hearing impairments (bottom) (from Erber, 1978, 1979d). Note differences between the groups in overall duration, syllable stress, syllable grouping, and pause location. Acoustic (or vibrotactile) instruction can be used to point out such intensity-feature distinctions to a profoundly hearing-impaired child, and thus can be used to guide speech development.

that is heard as a neighboring vowel or as a vowel of changing quality (diphthong). Investigators have reported a reduced range of both the first and second formants in vowels of hearing-impaired speakers (Angelocci, Kopp, & Holbrook, 1964; Monsen & Shaughnessy, 1978), indicating an inadequate range of tongue movement to clearly differentiate the vowels. The limited range of vowel articulation also may impair the intelligibility of adjacent consonants, whose correct identification often depends on appropriate vowel-formant transitions (Monsen, 1978).

Typical consonant-articulation problems exhibited by hearing-impaired children include: failure to distinguish between voiced/voiceless consonants, particularly the stops; misarticulation of certain speech sounds, particularly those with high-frequency components such as / s, ʃ /; and difficulty in producing smooth transitions in consonant-vowel or vowel-consonant syllables, in consonant blends, or in abutting consonants.

"linguistic" errors

Omission of an unstressed syllable or verb ending is relatively common in the spontaneous speech of many hearing-impaired children. Although these errors commonly are labeled as errors in expressive "language," they probably result from perceptual deficiencies. For example, verb endings, such as − s and − ing, and many other unstressed syllables typically are hard for a hearing-impaired child to hear or see when produced. Numerous children also misperceive unstressed prefixes and suffixes, plurals, pronouns, and prepositions, and so tend to use them improperly or not at all in their production of connected speech.

Clinical experience suggests that many of these speech errors can be minimized through careful and systematic instruction (Ling & Ling, 1978). This teaching may include the use of acoustic perception and imitation techniques as well as reliance on visual and tactile modeling.

general principles of acoustic speech instruction

rationale

In the preceding section, we have surveyed the common expressive errors of severely and profoundly hearing-impaired children. To correct these errors, a teacher should present acoustic models for imitation whenever possible (Beebe, 1953; Ling, 1976; Pollack, 1970). There are several specific reasons why acoustic modeling is important (Erber, 1980b).

For normally hearing people to communicate through speech, a correct series of *acoustic* events must be transmitted from talker to listener. Hearing people, in fact, *depend* on sound to perceive and process speech. If you were to regularly refer to the *acoustic* similarities and differences between your speech models and the child's imitations, then the child might be motivated to attend more carefully to these attributes and so to produce the *sounds* of speech more precisely. No visual, tactile, or manual method can convey this important concept so effectively.

The normal auditory system is better suited to perception of temporal events (as in speech) and to short-term memory recall (as in language processing) than is the visual system (Pickett, 1975). A child's auditory system (perhaps even one with a serious peripheral impairment) may be superior to the (intact) visual system for encoding, storing, and retrieving speech and speech-based language symbols—a hearing-impaired child who has learned to encode and recall language as a series of *acoustic* events may possess a more efficient method for speech processing and speech communication.

Finally, nonacoustic methods of speech feedback, correction, and instruction require special apparatus and/or the participation of a teacher. A

TABLE 9–1. Condensed version of a speech-skill inventory that can be used to specify a child's level of performance in speech production. Results are used to guide acoustic speech development and instruction.

---

1. Can child match vocal *duration* of vowels/words/phrases?
2. Can child produce vowels/words/phrases with appropriate *pitch* (intonation) with/without teacher's model?
3. Can child produce vowels/words/phrases/spontaneous speech with appropriate *voice quality*?
4. Can child produce *vowels/consonants* in isolation/in syllables/in repetitive syllables/in alternating syllables, in combination with other phonemes?
5. Can child produce acquired initial consonants/final consonants/vowels *in words* with/without teacher's model?
6. Can child produce appropriate durational patterns/pitch/voice quality/phonetic skills *in phrases and sentences* with/without teacher's model?

---

child's hearing aids and (impaired) ears are common feedback devices that are available to him or her at all times.

typical sequence

In general, the following steps are followed during acoustic speech instruction. The teacher develops an inventory of the child's speech production errors during conversation, as well as in a structured test situation (Table 9–1). The teacher also evaluates the child's capacity for auditory peception of speech. The typical child will be capable of perceiving certain acoustic distinctions between his or her own speech and that of the instructor, but will require further practice in perceiving certain other speech qualities (Chapter 2,4, and 5). To correct an error when a child produces improper speech or language, an acoustically oriented teacher will cover his or her mouth and repeatedly attempt to use sound as a stimulus before providing visible speech cues, exaggerating visible articulation, employing phonetic cues, or writing. Various useful acoustic strategies are available: repetition, exaggeration, intentional distortion, and verbal instruction (Erber & Greer, 1973). The teacher continually encourages the child to imitate acoustic speech models, and in time, the child learns self-monitoring and self-correction through auditory feedback.*

In sum, the teacher analyzes the child's perception and production for errors and notes their consistency, stimulates the child to talk so that the child's speech samples are available, acoustically models the correct speech and language, requests that the child imitate, judges the child's imitation,

---

*See Chapter 2, pages 25 to 27, for a detailed discussion of the role of perception in the modeling/imitation approach to speech instruction.

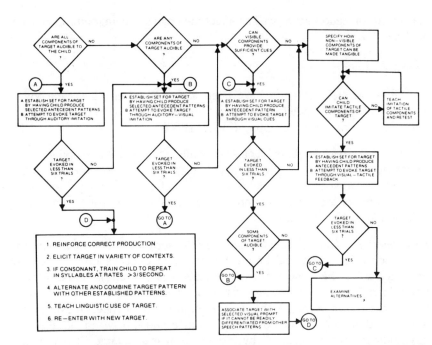

figure 9–2. Suggested sequence through which a teacher may employ a child's various sense modalities to teach speech production (from Ling & Ling, 1978).

tries various acoustic repetition and emphasis strategies, and allows visible or tactile articulatory cues if the child experiences persistent difficulty (Ling & Ling, 1978). (Figure 9–2).

obtaining a speech sample

How are speech samples obtained for analysis, modeling, and correction? Many children will speak when they simply want to tell or ask about something. Others must be stimulated in some way to produce an utterance. You may display an object and ask, "What is this?", write a word and request the child to say it, or ask a question ("How old are you?"). During either spontaneous or elicited speech, you should note articulation, voice, and/or language errors that are candidates for acoustic correction, *without* simultaneously lipreading the child.

After eliciting the speech and language, you are in a position to direct instruction. That is, if you obtain the child's utterance specifically for teaching purposes, you will feel relatively comfortable correcting speech. However, when the child speaks to you spontaneously, his or her purpose is to *communicate*, by sharing an internally generated idea. If you do not apply correction very cautiously in such instances, you may seriously disrupt the specific communication act as well as affect the child's general communication attitude.

special techniques

Five general strategies have been identified as effective in acoustic speech correction: repetition, exaggeration, intentional distortion, verbal instruction, and gestural prompting (Erber, 1980b).

Repetition. Basic situational factors may affect the child's perception of his or her own speech or that of your model (a lapse of attention, misperception due to reduced speech intensity or to noise in the room). Simple repetition of the model or the child's utterance may be sufficient to elicit an accurate imitation in these instances.

Exaggeration. Often, a speech element or a word will not produce a prominent (acoustic) perceptual image for the child because of distortion by hearing aid(s) or because of auditory limitations. For example, the child may not differentiate stress while producing the two syllables of the word *father*. You may attempt correction by exaggerating the differences in syllable intensity or duration (*fáð ɚ*). If the child omits a pause between clauses, you may indicate this pattern cue by modeling an exaggerated silence in the appropriate place to increase its perceptual prominence. Or if the child produces a word, phrase, or sentence with monotone pitch, you may model by exaggerating the magnitude of the correct intonation contour.

In addition, you might effectively use exaggeration in correcting a child's misarticulations, as when the child substitutes one consonant for another in his or her repertoire. For example, if a child produces / fid / for the word *feet*, you may cover your mouth and model the word for the child by exaggerating the intensity and duration of the final plosive burst. In the case of a vowel substitution or an error in vowel precision, try prolonging articulation of the vowel while the tongue is at the target position. Segments of diphthongs also may be exaggerated in a similar manner.

Whenever a child substitutes or omits a word (the zoo → *a* zoo) or morpheme (farmer → farm), produce the element with greater intensity and/or isolate it between brief pauses. For example, the phrase *in ... car* (incorrect) can be modeled for the child as *in ... a ... car* to stimulate correct production (Figure 9–3).

Intentional Distortion. The distortion technique is used mainly to elicit omitted phonemes; the object here is not to model correct acoustic patterns but to convince the child that it is the *sounds* of his or her speech that are important for perception by normally hearing people, and not the appearance of visible articulation. Once the child appreciates this concept, then you may model the correct production and request the child to imitate the speech segment while he or she receives its minimal feedback.

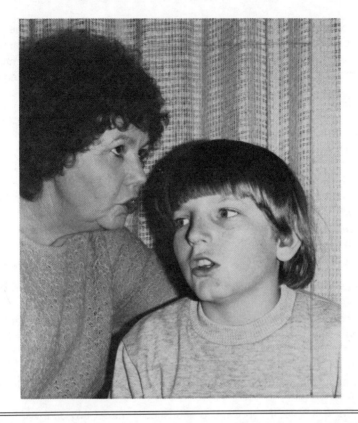

figure 9–3. A teacher uses the acoustic method to present a speech model to a hearing-impaired child.

Often a child may not be able to tell the difference between his or her production of a word with an omitted sound, and the teacher's production which includes the sound. How can acoustic modeling work in this case? Remember that an acoustic technique is appropriate only if the child seems capable of distinguishing acoustically between his or her incorrect production and the teacher's correct modeling of the speech sample. This is a reasonable minimum requirement for attempting acoustic correction. However, in some instances, when a child cannot make the distinction under normal conditions, you can apply intentional distortion to make the different acoustic qualities perceptually distinct. For example, you may be able to correct a child's omission or gross misarticulation of a stop or fricative (especially unvoiced phonemes, such as / p, t, f, s /) by moving the microphone very close to your (or the child's) mouth to create low-frequency turbulence from the breath stream (Schulte, 1978). The child usually can detect the resulting noise, which marks that point in the utterance where the particular speech sound (such as / s /) should occur. Later, although the child receives little or no auditory feedback when producing the sound correctly, he or she may recall the acoustic image of the teacher's distorted production. Correcting omission of an / s / might also be accomplished by cueing the child with an intentionally misarticulated / s / which is more like / ʃ / in quality. This lower-frequency sound often is audible to the child.

Verbal Instruction.   Teachers often provide a variety of graded suggestions, hints, and rules to guide the child in how to correct his or her own speech when the child fails to communicate (Calvert & Silverman, 1975). Some common verbal strategies are conveyed by the following: "I am listening carefully, but I still don't understand your speech" (general); "You forgot a sound in the last word" (more specific); or "You left out the / l / sound in the word *please*" (very specific). These suggestions, while not *acoustic* models themselves, instruct the child to modify the acoustic quality of his or her speech. Each suggestion not only provides a direction, but reminds the child that the way speech *sounds* is considered the most important factor.

Gestural Prompting.   Gestures, although they are not acoustic in nature, may be used to cue the child's attention to general acoustic events such as pitch change, pause, and stress, or to specific speech features such as voicing, nasality, stop, or frication. These gestures may be organized in the form of a phonetic cue system (Jenson, 1971; Schulte, 1978; Zaliouk, 1954) (Figure 9–4), or they may be more natural and spontaneous, as in body movements intended to convey rhythm and emphasis in speech (Guberina, 1967).

For example, if you want to acoustically model two different versions of a word for comparison—your *correct* production and the child's *incorrect* imitation—you might produce each sample while pointing to the person who produced it. You can easily indicate pitch change by raising or lowering your hand. You can suggest intensity errors by cupping your hand behind your ear (too soft) or by covering your ear (too loud). Many teachers also use natural gestures to indicate "repeat" (say it again), "stop," "listen," and so forth. All of these gestures refer to the *acoustic* nature of speech, although they, of course, produce no sound themselves.

additional strategies

A variety of additional strategies have proven useful in acoustic speech instruction in the classroom and clinic. For example, if the child succeeds in matching your acoustic speech model, you should acknowledge and reward the success to increase his or her confidence in hearing aids and ears for speech-monitoring. However, if the child continues to produce the error, apparently due to auditory limitations, you eventually must choose an alternative, more appropriate instructional strategy. Sometimes an auditory-visual compromise is effective, without resorting to obvious visible cueing,

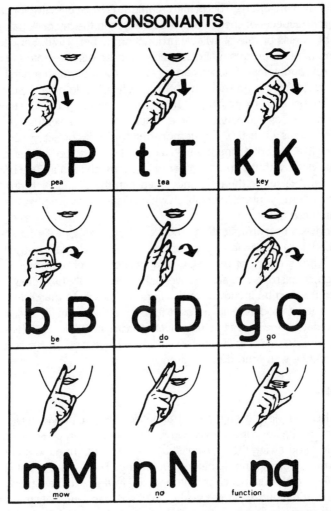

figure 9–4. The Phoneme-transmitting Manual System (PMS). Each hand sign can be used to convey phonetic and phonologic information to a hearing-impaired child during instruction in speech perception or production (from Schulte, 1978).

prompting, or articulatory modeling. Thus, if the child persists in producing / tip / for the word *keep*, you may simply uncover your mouth briefly to show the initial velar place of articulation, and then recover the mouth and model the entire word acoustically. That is, provide a relevant visible cue, but ultimately withdraw it, present the entire model *acoustically*, and then require the child to *listen*.

A profoundly hearing-impaired child can be taught to feel the output of a hand-held vibrator to compare the qualities of your speech model and his or her own imitations. This tactile technique is most effective for correcting those gross aspects of speech that are reflected in the intensity pattern, such as syllable stress or rate of syllable production (Erber, 1978; Schulte, 1978). But sometimes even minimal distinctions can be demonstrated in this way; some profoundly deaf children can be taught to distinguish a harsh (rough) or loud voice from a normal (smooth) or soft voice. In other instances, you may even be able to point out phonemic omissions or substitutions by modeling the correct pattern (for example / ǽp əℓ / versus / ǽ əℓ /; or / m u n / versus / b u d /). Try demonstrating the incorrect speech sample for the child and contrasting this with a correct vocal pattern. (This, of course, would be done with the mouth covered.) Ask the child to imitate both tactile qualities and describe the differences between the two speech productions. Feel the patterns yourself to establish which distinctions are possible tactually and which are not.

Nonvisual communication practice (as by telephone) is especially useful for convincing a child of the importance of *acoustically* correct speech. A child who is aware of the value of acoustic speech communication will allow you to disrupt a casual conversation repeatedly to model segments that you judge to be incorrect, and will try repeatedly to match the acoustic quality of your models. Still, an alert teacher will continually assess the situation to determine at what point to deemphasize acoustic speech instruction and resume an auditory-visual conversation. Decisions of this sort depend on experience with individual children.

caution

When employing any special acoustic cues or nonacoustic prompts described in the sections above, you should always complete the activity by gradually withdrawing the unusual supplementary information and returning to a normal acoustic model before continuing. That is, the intent should be to transfer the child's speech monitoring and imagery to the natural *acoustic* domain, rather than to increase the child's dependence on the substitute feedback that you provide. Ultimately, we want to help the child develop reliance on his or her hearing aids and (impaired) ears for self-monitoring and speech feedback.

summary

Both clinical observations and research findings have identified some of the perceptual errors that hearing-impaired children commonly experience, relating these findings to errors observed in their speech and language production. This chapter has explored some ways that a teacher can apply his or her knowledge of a child's auditory capabilities to correct the child's speech through acoustic modeling. A variety of special acoustically oriented strategies are available: repetition, exaggeration, intentional distortion, verbal instruction, gestural prompting, auditory-visual prompting, and tactile stimulation. The relative effectiveness of each of these methods will depend on each child's errors in speech production and on his or her auditory capabilities.

important communication factors

The development of speech perception abilities in a hearing-impaired child is a complicated and difficult task which depends on the successful interaction of numerous variables. The purpose of this final chapter is to emphasize the important role of the teacher, hearing clinician, or parent in helping a child to maximize use of his or her hearing capacity. A simple model of the communication chain will be presented to point out the many factors that can affect the ultimate success of an auditory training program, and ways in which a teacher can control these factors to enhance the child's communicative progress will be examined.

communication model

Consider eight major steps in the speech communication process (Figure 10–1):

1) The talker (teacher) forms the intended message in his or her brain.

2) This is converted to nerve impulses which cause the talker's articulators to produce the acoustic and optical components of speech. The talker monitors his or her speech through several feedback channels simultaneously (for example, auditory and tactile).

3) The coded acoustic and optical signals from the talker are transmitted through acoustic and optical environments, respectively.

THE COMMUNICATION PROCESS

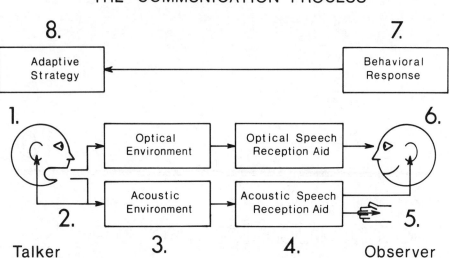

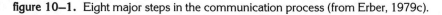

figure 10–1. Eight major steps in the communication process (from Erber, 1979c).

4) These signals may pass through speech perception aids (such as, an audio amplifier or eyeglasses) which make some dimensions of speech more prominent to the child.

5) The child's sensory systems receive the communication signals and convert them to nerve impulses which are conveyed to his or her brain.

6) These neural events are integrated and interpreted by the child on the basis of previously acquired experience and stored linguistic rules.

7) Aspects of the child's subsequent behavior indicate to the talker whether the child has perceived the intended message correctly.

8) If the child indicates that he or she has interpreted the message properly, then the talker may attempt to transmit a subsequent message, closely related to the first. If, however, the child indicates that he or she did not understand, then the talker may attempt to transmit the same message again, but this time perhaps in a somewhat different way.

Of all the factors involved in this process, probably the one that contributes most to a child's ultimate speech communication ability is his or her hearing capacity, that is, the child's potential for perceiving (amplified) speech through the ears, which depends on the condition of sensory and neural structures. Unfortunately, this seemingly critical component—the child's inherent hearing capacity—is a factor that *cannot* be modified; you may only work to maximize its use. It is recognized that the child also contributes several other personal characteristics which you cannot control—age, academic history, previous oral/aural experience, intelligence, and personality.

However, it is important to note, that the child (with his or her personal characteristics) forms only one or two segments of the entire speech communication chain. Most of the other vital links can be managed to an extent by you, the teacher. These include the effective use of available aids to speech perception (for example, an amplification system), careful elimination of potential distractors in the environment, and creative application of auditory training materials, methods, and strategies.

the teacher's responsibilities

Given some of the factors in the speech communication chain that tend to be the responsibility of the teacher, let us now consider how much each variable seems to contribute to successful speech perception by the child, and how the teacher can optimize communication in each case.

electronic aids to speech perception

With regard to the amplification system, it is mainly your responsibility to insure that your acoustic speech signal is amplified to an appropriate listening level and is delivered clearly and reliably to the child. This requires frequent and careful monitoring of batteries, switch-position and volume settings, earmolds, tubing, cords, and so on.* Obviously a weak battery or clogged earmold can make a hearing aid nonfunctional. Also routinely check the condition of the child's outer- and middle-ear, as the additional threshold shift caused by a conductive loss can seriously interfere with his or her auditory learning and communication (Osberger & Danaher, 1974).

The proper selection of a hearing aid, choice of gain setting, and earmold fit are extremely important factors in assuring the successful perception of speech. For moderately and severely hearing-impaired children, speech perception can be improved by more than 30 percent when adequately amplified acoustic cues from a hearing aid are provided along with visual cues from lipreading (Erber, 1971a). Conversely, a hearing-impaired child's auditory performance can fall 30 percent or more if the intensity of amplified speech decreases as little as 10 to 15 dB below the optimal listening

---

*Use an inexpensive stethoscope or a custom-made earmold to listen routinely to the child's hearing aid(s) for gross distortion, intermittency, or low gain. Be sure to listen also when you know the aid is functioning properly, so you will be able to recognize abnormal sounds. On a regular basis, you also should check for physical damage, such as clogged sound ports (microphone, earphone, tubing), loose or broken connectors, frayed cords, broken battery clips, defective switches, or a cracked case.

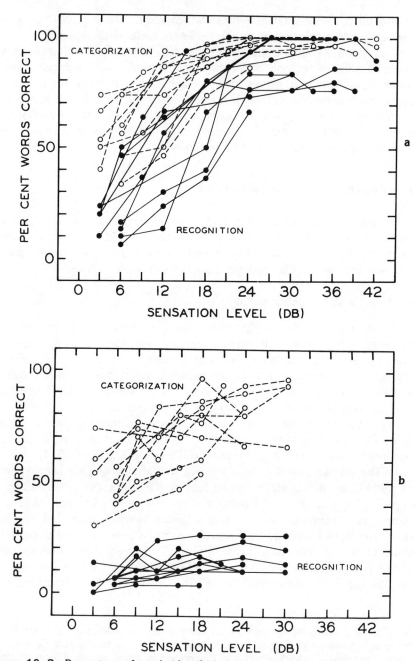

figure 10–2. Percentage of words identified and categorized into stress pattern by 10 severely hearing-impaired children (a) and by 10 profoundly hearing-impaired children (b). Their scores are shown as a function of acoustic stimulus level (dB re each child's speech-detection threshold) (from Erber & Witt, 1977). Note how scores increase for each group as the level of speech is increased.

level (Erber & Witt, 1977). Moreover, hearing-impaired children tend to make maximum use of acoustic cues only within a relatively narrow range of sound levels (Figure 10–2a). This will restrict how far you can move from the hearing aid and its microphone and still maintain adequate acoustic contact with the child during auditory training and communication.

A profoundly hearing-impaired child can identify the *stress patterns* of words much better when using his or her hearing aid at an appropriately high level than when listening near threshold (Erber & Witt, 1977) (Figure 10–2b). Reception of these acoustic cues can enhance lipreading perform-ance (auditory-visual perception) (Numbers & Hudgins, 1948), as well as the ability to self-monitor speech production. Obviously, the child can be deprived of potentially useful speech pattern information if his or her hearing aid is malfunctioning or if the amplified speech level is too low.

The greater the child's hearing loss, the greater the reliance on vision during auditory-visual perception of speech. Visual impairment among hear-ing-impaired children is relatively common (Levin & Erber, 1976), ranging between 20 to 40 percent of the children in special classes for the hearing impaired. Certain visual abnormalities can diminish speech perception from an estimated 30 percent decrement in lipreading performance for a child with 20/50 visual acuity to a 70 percent decrement for a child with 20/200 vision (Romano & Berlow, 1974). Be alert for common behavioral symptoms of visual disorder, such as crossed eyes, squinting, or complaints of head-ache, all of which may signal the need for referral to an ophthalmologist. For children who already use eyeglasses for vision correction, you must continually check for dirty or cracked lenses or loose frames which can impede visual, and thus auditory-visual, perception. In cases where a child is known to have a vision disorder which is *not* correctable (such as reduced visual fields or color blindness), you can accommodate to that child's special visual and auditory-visual needs by providing optimal seating, direct illumi-nation, large type, or special color contrast on learning materials.

classroom environment

acoustic factors

Regarding the acoustic environment of the classroom, noise and re-verberation in close proximity to the hearing aid and its microphone can have serious detrimental effects on speech communication between a teacher and child. These negative changes in auditory or auditory-visual perception can be moderately large (30 to 50 percent) under very poor acoustic con-ditions where the speech-to-noise ratio is low (Erber, 1971a) or when room reverberation (echo) is high (Borrild, 1978; Olsen, 1977). If you are always careful to be near the hearing aid microphone while talking, you can easily minimize the disruptive effects of poor acoustic surroundings (Figure 10–3).

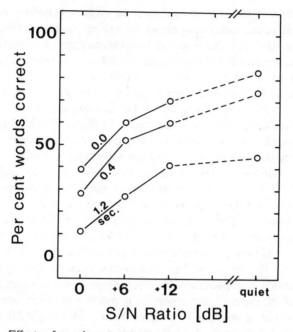

figure 10–3. Effects of reverberation time and room noise on auditory identification of words through hearing aids by 12 moderately hearing-impaired children (from Finitzo-Hieber & Tillman, 1978).

Moreover, you should be particularly attentive to unnecessary noise produced by the children themselves and suppress these sounds as they are most likely to interfere with communication in a group. It is quite common for children to generate noise in a classroom by talking, coughing, kicking furniture, dropping books, clicking pens, or slamming doors. Try to be especially sensitive to these potential distractors and explain why it is important for everyone to be quiet when someone is talking and others are listening.

Certain other noises, however, may be the result of architectural or construction errors. Doors and windows may not close or isolate areas properly, allowing unwanted sound from a hallway or playground to enter the classroom. Often, the level of intruding noise can be reduced by installing special rubber or wool felt seals to minimize sound leakage. If, for example, a classroom is located near a rhythm and music room in which high sound levels are generated, this noise-transmission problem can sometimes be solved by relocating the classroom or isolating the sound sources within that special-purpose room. High levels of impact or scraping noise usually are reduced simply by installing carpet on the floor. In other rooms where children must communicate to learn, noise may be produced as an integral part of the associated activity, as, for example, in a cooking class or a woodworking shop. In these cases, excessive noise is lessened somewhat by applying rubber mats to work surfaces, by using wood or plastic tools and utensils wherever possible, and by restricting vibrating equipment such as an electric drill or blender to a designated area of the classroom.

optical factors

It is well known that the optical environment, such as the angles of the talker's mouth and incident light, the distance between the teacher and child, and the level of illumination all can affect a child's visual perception of speech through lipreading (Erber, 1971b, 1974a) thus affecting his or her combined auditory-visual perception of speech. Increasing angle and increasing distance both have been shown to produce decrements of from 10 to 20 percent in word recognition through lipreading under extreme conditions (such as angles greater than 45° or distances between 5 and 20 meters). On the other hand, reduction in overall light level does not seem to decrease visual perception of speech to such a great extent (5 to 10 percent). To minimize eye fatigue, you should attempt to create as diffuse an optical environment as possible—a softly glowing room rather than a sharply glaring one. This involves eliminating extreme contrasts in brightness and highly reflective surfaces (for example, exposed light sources, mirrors, chrome doorknobs or window handles, and jewelry). Although these are optical distractors, they can easily capture a child's attention and so reduce his or her awareness of acoustic input during auditory instruction.

The arrangement of materials beside and behind the teacher also can have an important effect on auditory-visual communication. Teachers have reported that a young child's visual attention may shift from the talker's face to colorful pictures or toys in the vicinity. Classroom visitors also are a common distraction. Although the disruptive effect in these cases cannot easily be quantified, you can plan the arrangement of furniture and displays to minimize optical competition in the teaching environment. In fact, a teacher usually has considerable control over the optical environment in the classroom. To optimize optical conditions for auditory-visual perception of speech face the primary source of light, keep the viewing distances short and the desk-chair arrangements compact, and eliminate potentially distracting objects and surfaces from the child's visual field.

clarity of speech

The clarity of your speech is a function of the positions, movements, and timing of your articulators in the process of communicating a message. A child's ability to perceive your message accurately will depend on the degree to which the acoustic and optical components of your speech signal match his or her internally stored set of spoken language patterns. You may inadvertently obscure your speech either acoustically, by using an excessively high voice pitch or low intensity, or optically, by simply possessing large teeth or a small, immobile mouth. And, if you articulate rapidly or imprecisely, children may misperceive your speech through both listening and lipreading. In fact, formal comparisons between naive speakers and those experienced in communicating orally with hearing-impaired children have shown that differences as great as 20 to 30 percent can occur in vowel, consonant, and word intelligibility through lipreading (Pesonen, 1968; Pintner, Eisenson & Stanton, 1941). In addition, male talkers tend to be somewhat more intelligible acoustically than females (Pascoe, 1975), probably because of their lower voice pitches and also the lower frequencies of their vowel formants. Significant differences can exist even in the acoustic *intensity patterns* of the speech of different talkers (Knudsen, 1928).

As mentioned, moderately large differences in speech clarity (and thus intelligibility) are quite common between experienced and inexperienced teachers. Surprisingly, considerable differences have also been observed in acoustic speech clarity between teachers with *similar* amounts of classroom experience, perhaps due to anatomical differences in their articulators, or to variation in awareness of the factors that optimize communication.* Still, it is possible to improve your acoustic speech intelligibility through specific training and feedback (Black, 1956). In general, both acoustic and optical speech clarity can be enhanced by slightly slowing speech and carefully articulating with an effort to provide moderate emphasis to each syllable. Unfortunately, a set of general principles and practical methods to create uniformly high speech clarity, or intelligibility, among all teachers of hearing-impaired children has not yet been developed.

As a minimum requirement, however, teachers, hearing specialists, and parents always should be conscious of their speech. Additionally, as a teacher, you should constantly encourage hearing-impaired pupils to inform you if: 1) your speech is too loud, distorting the acoustic speech patterns (they usually will report this); 2) your speech is too soft, rendering critical elements of speech inaudible (some children will fail to report this, and substitute lipreading instead); 3) you are talking too fast, taxing their short-term memories (some children will not recognize this as a source of their perceptual difficulties). A child's successful oral communication and auditory learning depends on the acoustic clarity of your speech. In the absence of this clarity, the child may learn to depend instead on visible articulations, gestures, or situational cues for meaning. Therefore, constantly experiment with different acoustic speech levels or rates to determine which ones enhance your intelligibility and which ones cause difficulty.

Several instruments are available to analyze some physical correlates of your speech clarity. For example, it may be useful to record your voice

---

*These differences in intelligibility may be apparent only to someone with impaired hearing—the children in your class.

for basic spectrographic analysis, that is, fundamental voice pitch, vowel-formant frequencies, degree of breathiness or nasality, and so forth. In addition, you can make use of videotape apparatus for self-observation of your audible and visible speech patterns, as well as visible facial or gestural cues that you provide during auditory training. You may even listen to your own speech through special filters, distortion devices, or vibrotactile apparatus to experience, through simulation, the perceptual effects of your pupils' hearing losses (Erber, 1976; Erber & Zeiser, 1974; Gagné & Erber, 1980).*

message structure and content

The teacher's choice of the spoken message can strongly influence auditory-visual speech perception by a hearing-impaired child. This effect is greatest when the child has limited vocabulary, poor knowledge of language, or little experience with typical conversational sequences. Certain speech items are relatively easy to identify. Others are inherently difficult to perceive accurately—even for a child with an acquired hearing loss who possesses a large vocabulary and a well-developed knowledge of language. For example, it is well known that the stress pattern of a word can influence its intelligibility. Spondees (two stressed syllables) tend to be more intelligible than trochees (one stressed, one unstressed syllable), which in turn are easier to identify than monosyllabic words. This word effect occurs both for auditory and visual perception of speech (Erber, 1971b). Short, simple sentences of familiar form tend to be more intelligible than long, complex sentences (Clouser, 1976).

Perception of speech is enhanced with the inclusion of phonemes, words, or phrases that you know are distinctive.**That is, you can carefully assemble a sentence to increase its auditory intelligibility to a hearing-impaired child. A child also is more likely to understand the sentence if it is appropriate to the situational context. If you are careless, and do not plan sentence construction accordingly, the child may have unnecessary difficulty. Thus, the structure and content of your spoken messages can make the difference between auditory comprehension and perceptual confusion (a difference of up to 100 percent), especially for a hearing-impaired child with incomplete knowledge of language.

---

*You can crudely simulate a severe hearing impairment by listening to recorded speech through a 500 Hz low-pass filter (but see Gagné & Erber, 1980), and a profound hearing loss by feeling the same speech signal through a vibrator. In the latter case, your hand should be sealed in a small sound-isolation chamber, and your ears should be isolated further in muff-type ear protectors (Erber, 1976).

**See Chapter 2 and Chapter 4, page 61 (footnote).

TABLE 10–1. Remedial strategies commonly used by teachers to clarify oral/aural communication with hearing-impaired children. Examples are given to illustrate the four main types of instructional behavior (from Erber & Greer, 1973).

A. *Repetition*
1. Repetition of a word (R-w)
   T: Where do we eat?
   C: Food.
   T: Where?
2. Repetition of a phrase (R-p)
   T: Put the ball on the table.
   C: (Puts the ball on box)
   T: On the table.
3. Repetition of a sentence (R-s)
   T: What do you wear on your feet?
   C: (No response)
   T: What do you wear on your feet?

B. *Emphasis* (often associated with repetition)
1. Increased vocal effort (E-e)
   T: Please stand in the circle.
   C: (Stands in wrong place)
   T: *Please stand in the circle.* (sentence) Please stand *in the circle.* (phrase) Please stand in the *circle.* (word)
2. Emphasis through prosody or intonation (E-p/i)
   T: Why do the animals look so happy?
   C: (No response)
   T: Why do the animals look so happy?
3. Exaggerated oral/facial articulation (E-a)
   T: Where did the cats go?
   C: (No response)
   T: Where did the c---ats go?

C. *Structural Change*
1. Variation in word order (SC-o)
   T: Where are the boys going?
   C: Tomorrow.
   T: The boys are going where?
2. Word/phrase addition (SC-a)
   T: The children were tired.
   C: What?
   T: The children were very tired.

3. Simplification through word/phrase deletion; subject and verb of independent clause retained (SC-d)
   T: How do you feel about that?
   C: (No response)
   T: How do you feel?
4. Simplification through word/phrase substitution (SC-s)
   T: The boys picked up all of the toys in the room.
   C: What?
   T: The boys picked up everything.
5. Clause inversion (SC-i)
   T: If we are late, we will miss the bus.
   C: I don't understand.
   T: We will miss the bus if we are late.
6. Complex change (SC-c)
   T: What was left after she bought the apples?
   C: (No response)
   T: How much money did she have?

D. *Supplementary Information*
1. Verbal prompt (SI-v)
   T: Where is your coat?
   C: (No response)
   T: On the floor? At home? In your locker?
2. Reference to written material (SI-w)
   T: Who knows what *evaporation* means?
   C: (No response)
   T: (Writes *evaporation* on the chalkboard)
3. Picture/object prompt (SI-p/o)
   T: Whose shoe is this?
   C: (No response)
   T: (Holds up shoe)
4. Gestural cue (SI-g)
   T: Put on your earphones.
   C: (No response)
   T: (points to ears)

methods and strategies

Teachers use numerous methods and strategies, both in their initial attempts to communicate aurally and also in remedial attempts if earlier trials have failed. Many instructional techniques seem to be especially useful, such as, contriving daily experiences to stimulate classroom discussion (Golf, 1974), motivating children by creating a need to communicate orally (Moog, 1975), and emphasizing individual or small-group instruction (Pollack, 1974). Helpful clarification strategies that teachers frequently employ include repetition of all or part of a sentence, emphasis (exaggeration) of all or part of a sentence, modification of vocabulary or language, and use of information that may be presented through speech, writing, or tangible objects (Erber & Greer, 1973) (Table 10–1).

the child's response is the teacher's stimulus

As explained in Chapters 3,5, and 7, many teachers employ a type of "adaptive" instruction (Erber, 1977a) in which each communication event is considered an informal auditory test at particular stimulus and response levels (Chapter 3, Figure 3–5). The teacher analyzes the child's recent responses to determine whether he or she is functioning adequately at the chosen level of auditory communication. At any time, the teacher may decide to increase or decrease the complexity of the task, depending upon whether the child has experienced success or difficulty with recent auditory requirements. In addition, these choices are influenced by the intent: 1) to transmit information accurately through acoustic messages constructed for high intelligibility; or 2) to expand the child's knowledge of acoustically encoded language by using vocabulary and syntax which may be only marginally familiar.

The role and effectiveness of specific teaching strategies in the auditory instruction of hearing-impaired children is not at all clear. Certainly, it is important to choose instructional methods that maintain the child's interest, motivation, and listening attitude and that provide continuity between teaching units. Conscious use of elaborate communication strategies, however, seems much less necessary for mildly and moderately hearing-impaired children than for children who are severely or profoundly hearing impaired. Those with mild and moderate impairments often accurately perceive even casually spoken messages through audition or combined auditory-visual modes. They respond correctly, and consequently their teachers and parents tend to provide frequent opportunities for auditory practice and reinforcement.

On the other hand, severely and profoundly hearing-impaired children, may misperceive acoustic messages on the first or second try, respond incorrectly or not at all, and get discouraged during difficult auditory communication tasks. Moreover, they may resort to supplementing acoustic speech information by attending to visible gestures and situational cues. Most teachers agree that carefully directed, systematic listening practice is necessary to prevent, or at least minimize, these consequences of communication difficulty experienced during critical points in a child's auditory development.

A severely or profoundly hearing-impaired child's communicative progress strongly depends on the opportunity to repeatedly experience *success* in auditory speech perception. It takes a skillful teacher to accomplish this goal aurally—through manipulation of spoken messages, response choices, situational contexts, speech qualities, and verbal prompts—without resorting excessively to lipreading cues, gestures, or other forms of visible communication.

Usually, it is not necessary for teachers and parents to adopt extraordinary methods and special strategies for enhancing the auditory development of a mildly or moderately hearing-impaired child, provided that the child listens through functioning hearing aids and attends to a nearby talker in a relatively quiet environment, and that the talker uses moderate care in speech production. In contrast, these same minimal conditions of hearing aid function, classroom environment, and careful articulation do not seem sufficient to insure rapid development of auditory speech (and language) perception abilities in a severely or profoundly hearing-impaired child. Instead, in such cases, the teacher must be able to present spoken messages carefully, apply auditory instruction methods creatively, and select confidently from a repertoire of remedial strategies when communication difficulty occurs. If you apply appropriate strategies when needed, you can help the child to succeed and to develop as an auditory communicator.

summary and conclusion

Numerous variables influence aural communication between a teacher and a hearing-impaired child. You cannot easily modify the child's hearing capacity, intellect, or personality; these attributes form the raw material for development. But many other factors are primarily your responsibility:

1) the proper use of functioning amplification equipment;
2) the quality of the acoustic and optical environments;
3) the content and structure of your intended spoken message;
4) the clarity of your audible and visible speech articulation;
5) the creative use of instructional methods and materials;
6) the effective application of remedial auditory communication strategies.

If you are careful to optimize all of the conditions under which auditory instruction occurs, then the child will learn to listen and to perceive speech with maximum ease. Helping a specific hearing-impaired child develop his or her auditory performance to capacity is not always an easy task; to succeed, you will need to express a positive attitude, expend considerable energy, receive recognition and praise for the effort, and feel the pride of accomplishment.

When these questions are asked, how will you answer? . . .

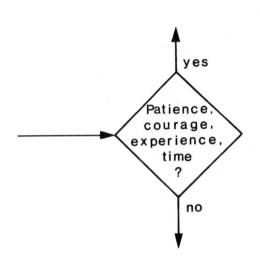

references

Alich, G. W. Language communication by lipreading. In *Proceedings of the International Conference on Oral Education of the Deaf.* Washington, DC: A.G. Bell Association for the Deaf, 1967.

Angelocci, A.A., Kopp, G.A., & Holbrook, A. The vowel formants of deaf and normal-hearing eleven- to fourteen-year-old boys. *Journal of Speech and Hearing Disorders,* 1964, *29,* 156–170.

Argila, C.A. *A computer simulation of lipreading.* Unpublished Ph.D. dissertation, University of Santo Tomas, Philippines, 1978.

Asp, C.W. The Verbo-Tonal Method as an alternative to present auditory training techniques. In J.W. Wingo & G.F. Holloway, (Eds.), *An appraisal of speech pathology and audiology.* Springfield, IL: Thomas, 1973.

Ballweber, D., & Jackson, P.L. The relationship between word and stress pattern recognition ability and hearing level in hearing-impaired young adults. Paper presented at the A.G. Bell Association for the Deaf Convention, St. Louis, MO, 1978.

Beebe, H. *A guide to help the severely hard of hearing child.* Basel/New York: Karger, 1953.

Bennett, C. W., & Ling, D. Effects of voiced-voiceless discrimination training upon articulation of hearing-impaired children. *Language and Speech,* 1977, *20,* 287–294.

Black, J.W. *Voice communication: A bibliographic and annotated summary of ten years of research.* (Office of Naval Research, Contract N6onr–22525, NR 145–993) Columbus, OH: Ohio State University, 1956.

Boothroyd, A. The discrimination by partially hearing children of frequency distorted speech. *International Audiology,* 1967, *6,* 136–145.

Boothroyd, A. Statistical theory of the speech discrimination score. *Journal of the Acoustical Society of America* 1968, *43,* 362–367.

Boothroyd, A. *Auditory training handbook.* Northampton, MA: Clarke School for the Deaf, 1971.

185

Boothroyd, A. Sensory aids research project—Clarke School for the Deaf. In G. Fant (Ed.), *Speech communication ability and profound deafness*. Washington, DC: A.G. Bell Association for the Deaf, 1972.

Boothroyd, A. Influence of residual hearing on speech perception and speech production by hearing-impaired children. Paper presented at the annual convention of the American Speech-Language-Hearing Association, Houston, TX, 1976.

Boothroyd, A. Speech perception and sensorineural hearing loss. In M. Ross & T.G. Giolas (Eds), *Auditory management of hearing-impaired children*. Baltimore: University Park Press, 1978.

Boothroyd, A., & Cawkwell, S. Vibrotactile thresholds in pure tone audiometry. *Acta Oto-Laryngologica*, 1970, *69*, 381–387.

Boothroyd, A., & Decker, M. Control of voice pitch by the deaf. *Audiology*, 1972, *11*, 343–353.

Borrild, K. Classroom acoustics. In M. Ross & T.G. Giolas (Eds.), *Auditory management of hearing-impaired children*. Baltimore: University Park Press, 1978.

Braida, L.D., Durlach, N.I., Lippmann, R.P., Hicks, B.L., Rabinowitz, W.M., & Reed, C. M. Hearing aids—a review of past research on linear amplification, amplitude compression, and frequency lowering. *ASHA Monograph* No. 19, 1979.

Briskey, R.J., & Sinclair, J. The importance of low frequency amplification in deaf children. *Audecibel*, 1966, *15*, 7–20.

Butt, D.S., & Chreist, F.M. A speechreading test for young children. *The Volta Review*, 1968, *70*, 225–239.

Byers, V.W. Initial consonant intelligibility by hearing-impaired children. *Journal of Speech and Hearing Research*, 1973, *16*, 48–55.

Calvert, D.R., Speech sound duration and the surd-sonant error. *The Volta Review*, 1962, *64*, 401–403.

Calvert, D.R., & Silverman, S.R. *Speech and deafness*. Washington, DC: A.G. Bell Association for the Deaf, 1975.

Castle, D.L. Telephone training for the deaf. *The Volta Review*, 1977, *79*, 373–378.

Castle, D.L. Telephone communication for the hearing impaired: Methods and equipment. *Journal of the Academy of Rehabilitative Audiology*, 1978, *11*, 91–104.

Clark, G.M., Pyman, B.C., & Bailey, Q.R. The surgery for multiple-electrode cochlear implantations. *Journal of Laryngology and Otology*, 1979, *93*, 215–223.

Clouser, R.A. The effect of vowel consonant ratio and sentence length on lipreading ability. *American Annals of the Deaf*, 1976, *121*, 513–518.

Connors, S., & McPherson, D.L. A vibrotactile training program for the deaf using a single vibrator. In D.L. McPherson (Ed.), *Advances in prosthetic devices for the deaf: A technical workshop*. Rochester, NY: NTID, Rochester Institute of Technology, 1979.

Conrad, R. Profound deafness as a psycholinguistic problem. In G. Fant (Ed.), *Speech communication ability and profound deafness*. Washington, DC: A.G. Bell Association for the Deaf, 1972.

Craig, H.B., Craig, W.N., & Sehlin, C. *Pittsburgh Auditory Test*. Pittsburgh: Western Pennsylvania School for the Deaf, 1975.

Craig, H.B., Sins, V.A., & Rossi, S.L. *Your child's hearing aid*. Lake Oswego, OR: Dormac, Inc., 1976.

Cramer, K.D. & Erber, N.P. A spondee-recognition test for young hearing-impaired children. *Journal of Speech and Hearing Disorders*, 1974, *39*, 304–311.

Dale, D.M.C. *Applied audiology for children.* Springfield, IL: Charles C. Thomas 1962.

Danaher, E.M., & Pickett, J.M. Some masking effects produced by low-frequency vowel formants in persons with sensorineural hearing loss. *Journal of Speech and Hearing Research,* 1975, *18,* 261–271.

DeFilippo, C.L. Tactile aids for the deaf: Design and evaluation strategies. In D.L. McPherson (Ed.) *Advances in prosthetic devices for the deaf: A technical workshop,* Rochester, NY: NTID, Rochester Institute of Technology, 1979.

DeFilippo, C.L. Memory for articulated sequences and lipreading performance of deaf observers. *The Volta Review* 1982, *84,* 134–146.

DeFilippo, C.L., & Scott, B.L. A method for training and evaluating the reception of ongoing speech. *Journal of the Acoustical Society of America,* 1978, *63,* 1186–1192.

DiCarlo, L . Some relationships between frequency discrimination and speech reception performance. *Journal of Auditory Research,* 1962, *2,* 37–49.

Doehring, D.G. Picture-sound association in deaf children. *Journal of Speech and Hearing Research* 1968, *11,* 49–62.

Edson, S. *The acoustic approach to speech correction.* Independent study, Central Institute for the Deaf, Washington University, St. Louis, MO, 1978.

Erber, N.P., Auditory and audiovisual reception of words in low-frequency noise by children with normal hearing and by children with impaired hearing. *Journal of Speech and Hearing Research,* 1971, *14,* 496–512. (a)

Erber, N.P. Effects of distance on the visual perception of speech. *Journal of Speech and Hearing Research,* 1971, *14,* 848–857. (b)

Erber, N.P. Auditory, visual, and auditory-visual recognition of consonants by children with normal and impaired hearing. *Journal of Speech and Hearing Research,* 1972, *15,* 413–422. (a)

Erber, N.P. Speech envelope cues as an acoustic aid to lipreading for profoundly deaf children. *Journal of the Acoustical Society of America,* 1972, *51,* 1224–1227. (b)

Erber, N.P. Body-baffle and real-ear effects in the selection of hearing aids for deaf children. *Journal of Speech and Hearing Disorders,* 1973, *38,* 224–231.

Erber, N.P. Effects of angle, distance, and illumination on visual reception of speech by profoundly deaf children. *Journal of Speech and Hearing Research,* 1974, *17,* 99–112. (a)

Erber, N.P. Lip-reading skills. In R.E. Stark (Ed.), *Sensory capabilities of hearing-impaired children.* Baltimore: University Park Press, 1974. (b)

Erber, N.P. Pure-tone thresholds and word recognition abilities of hearing-impaired children. *Journal of Speech and Hearing Research,* 1974, *17,* 194–202. (c)

Erber, N.P. Visual perception of speech by deaf children: Recent developments and continuing needs. *Journal of Speech and Hearing Disorders,* 1974, *39,* 178–185. (d)

Erber, N.P., Auditory-visual perception of speech. *Journal of Speech and Hearing Disorders,* 1975, *40,* 481–492.

Erber, N.P. The use of audio tape cards in auditory training for hearing-impaired children. *The Volta Review* 1976, *78,* 209–218.

Erber, N.P. Developing materials for lipreading evaluation and instruction. *The Volta Review,* 1977, *79,* 35–42. (a)

Erber, N.P. Evaluating speech-perception ability in hearing-impaired children. In F.H. Bess (Ed.), *Childhood deafness.* New York: Grune & Stratton, 1977. (b)

Erber, N.P. Vibratory perception by deaf children. *International Journal of Rehabilitation Research,* 1978, *1,* 27–37.

Erber, N.P. An approach to evaluating auditory speech perception ability. *The Volta Review,* 1979, *81,* 17–24. (a)

Erber, N.P. Auditory-visual perception of speech with reduced optical clarity. *Journal of Speech and Hearing Research,* 1979, *22,* 212–223. (b)

Erber, N.P., Optimizing speech communication in the classroom. In A. Simmons-Martin & D.R. Calvert (Eds.), *Parent-infant intervention: Communication disorders.* New York: Grune & Stratton, 1979. (c)

Erber, N.P. Speech perception by profoundly hearing-impaired children. *Journal of Speech and Hearing Disorders,* 1979, *44,* 255–270. (d)

Erber, N.P., Auditory evaluation and training of hearing-impaired children. *Journal of the National Student Speech and Hearing Association,* 1980, *8,* 6–18. (a)

Erber, N.P. Speech correction through use of acoustic models. In J.D. Subtelny (Ed.), *Speech assessment and speech improvement for the hearing impaired.* Washington, DC: A.G. Bell Association for the Deaf, 1980. (b)

Erber, N.P. Use of the Auditory Numbers Test to evaluate speech perception abilities of hearing-impaired children. *Journal of Speech and Hearing Disorders,* 1980, *45,* 527–532. (c)

Erber, N.P., & Alencewicz, C.M. Audiologic evaluation of deaf children. *Journal of Speech Hearing Disorders,* 1976, *41,* 256–267.

Erber, N.P., & Greer, C.W. Communication strategies used by teachers at an oral school for the deaf. *The Volta Review,* 1973, *75,* 480–485.

Erber, N.P., & Hirsh, I.J. Auditory training. In H. Davis & R.S. Silverman (Eds.), *Hearing and deafness* (4th ed.). New York: Holt, Rinehart, and Winston, 1978.

Erber, N.P., & McMahan, D.A. Effects of sentence context on recognition of words through lipreading by deaf children. *Journal of Speech and Hearing Research,* 1976, *19,* 112–119.

Erber, N.P., & Witt, L.H. Effects of stimulus intensity on speech perception by deaf children. *Journal of Speech and Hearing Disorders,* 1977, *42,* 271–278.

Erber, N.P., & Zeiser, M.L. Classroom observation under conditions of simulated profound deafness. *The Volta Review,* 1974, *76,* 352–360.

Ewing, I.R., & Ewing, A.W.G. *New opportunities for deaf children.* London: University of London Press, Ltd., 1961.

Fifield, D.B., Earnshaw, R., & Smither, M. A new ear impression technique to prevent acoustic feedback with high powered hearing aids. *The Volta Review,* 1980, *82,* 33–39.

Finitzo-Hieber, T., & Tillman, T.W. Room acoustics effects on monosyllabic word discrimination ability for normal and hearing-impaired children. *Journal of Speech and Hearing Research,* 1978, *21,* 440–458.

Fisher, C.G. Confusions among visually perceived consonants. *Journal of Speech and Hearing Research,* 1968, *11,* 796–804.

Fletcher, H. *Speech and hearing.* New York: Van Nostrand, 1929.

Gagne, J.P., & Erber, N.P. Simulation of severe sensorineural hearing impairment. Paper presented at the Annual Convention of the A.G. Bell Association for the Deaf, Houston, TX, 1980.

Gault, R.H. Touch as a substitute for hearing in the interpretation and control of speech. *Archives of Otolaryngology*, 1926, *3*, 121–135. (a)

Gault, R.H. The interpretation of speech by tactual and visual impression. *Archives of Otolaryngology*, 1926, *4*, 228–239. (b)

Gault, R.H. On the interpretation of speech sounds by means of their tactual correlates. *Annals of Otology, Rhinology, and Laryngology*, 1926, *35*, 1050–1063. (c)

Gault, R.H. On the identification of certain vowel and consonantal elements in words by their tactual qualities and by their visual qualities as seen by the lipreader. *Journal of Abnormal Psychology*, 1927, *22*, 33–39.

Gault, R.H. On the extension of the use of the sense of touch in relation to the training and education of the deaf. *American Annals of the Deaf*, 1928, *73*, 134–146. (a)

Gault, R.H. Interpretation of spoken language when the feel of speech supplements vision of the speaking face. *The Volta Review*, 1928, *30*, 379–386. (b)

Gault, R.H. A partial analysis of the effects of tactual-visual stimulation by spoken language. *Journal of the Franklin Institute*, 1930, *209*, 437–458.

Gengel, R.W. Practice effects in frequency discrimination by hearing-impaired children. *Journal of Speech and Hearing Research*, 1969, *12*, 847–856.

Gengel, R.W. On the reliability of discrimination-performance in persons with sensorineural hearing impairment using a closed-set. *Journal of Auditory Research*, 1973, *13*, 97–100.

Gengel, R.W., Pascoe, D., & Shore, I. A frequency-response procedure for evaluating and selecting hearing aids for severely hearing-impaired children. *Journal of Speech and Hearing Disorders*, 1971, *36*, 341–353.

Gold, T. Speech production in hearing-impaired children. *Journal of Communication Disorders*, 1980, *13*, 397–418.

Goldstein, M.A. *Problems of the deaf.* St. Louis: The Laryngoscope Press, 1933.

Goldstein, M.A. *The acoustic method.* St. Louis: The Laryngoscope Press, 1939.

Golf, H.R. Speech through auditory training. In *Report of the Proceedings of the 44th Meeting of the Convention of American Instructors of the Deaf.* Washington, DC: U.S. Government Printing Office, 1970.

Golf, H.R. Strategies for teaching 4 to 8 year olds. In *Proceedings of the 46th Meeting of the Convention of American Instructors of the Deaf.* Washington, DC: U.S. Government Printing Office, 1974.

Grammatico, L. Learning to process auditory information. In C. Griffiths (Ed.), *Proceedings of International Conference on Auditory Techniques.* Springfield, IL: Charles C. Thomas, 1974.

Groht, M.A. *Natural language for deaf children.* Washington, DC: A.G. Bell Association for the Deaf, 1958.

Guberina, P. Verbotonal method and its application to the rehabilitation of the deaf. *Proceedings of the International Congress on Education of the Deaf.* Washington, DC: U.S. Government Printing Office, 1964.

Guberina, P. The use of phonetic rhythm in the verbotonal system. *International Congress on Oral Education of the Deaf*, Washington, DC: A.G. Bell Association for the Deaf, 1967.

Guttman, N., & Nelson, J.R. An instrument that creates some artificial speech spectra for the severely hard of hearing. *American Annals of the Deaf*, 1968, *113*, 295–302.

Hack, Z.C., & Erber, N.P. Auditory, visual and auditory-visual perception of vowels by hearing-impaired children. *Journal of Speech and Hearing Research*, 1982, *25*, 100–107.

Hopkins, L.A., & Hudgins, C.V. The relationship between degree of deafness and response to acoustic training. *Volta Review*, 1953, *55*, 32–35.

House, W.F. Cochlear implants. *Annals of Otology, Rhinology and Laryngology*, 1976, *85* (Suppl. 27), 1–93.

Hudgins, C.V. A rationale for acoustic training. *The Volta Review*, 1948, *50*, 484–490.

Hudgins, C.V. A method of appraising the speech of the deaf. *The Volta Review*, 1949, *51*, 597–601; 638.

Hudgins, C.V. Auditory training: Its possibilities and limitations. *The Volta Review*, 1954, *56*, 339–349.

Hudgins, C.V., & Numbers, F.C. An investigation of intelligibility of the speech of the deaf. *Genetic Psychology Monographs*, 1942, *25*, 289–392.

Huizing, H.C. Deaf-mutism—modern trends in treatment and prevention. In L. Rüedi(Ed.), *Advances in oto-rhino-laryngology*. Basel, Switzerland: Karger, 1959.

Jeffers, J., & Barley, M. *Speechreading (lipreading)*. Springfield IL: Charles C Thomas, 1971.

Jenson, P.M. The relationship of speechreading and speech. In L.E. Connor(Ed.), *Speech for the deaf child: Knowledge and use*. Washington, DC: A.G. Bell Association for the Deaf, 1971.

Johanssen, B. The use of the transposer for the management of the deaf child. *International Audiology*, 1966, *5*, 362–372.

Kalikow, D.N., Stevens, K.N., & Elliott, L.L. Development of a test of speech intelligibility in noise using sentence materials of controlled word predictability. *Journal of the Acoustic Society of America*, 1977, *61*, 1337–1351.

Killian, M.C. Earmold options for wideband hearing aids. *Journal of Speech and Hearing Disorders*, 1981, *46*, 10–20.

Kirman, J.H. Tactile communication of speech: A review and an analysis. *Psychology Bulletin* 1973, *80*, 54–74.

Knudsen, V.O. "Hearing" with the sense of touch. *Journal of Genetic Psychology*, 1928, *1*, 320–352.

Kringlebotn, M. Experiments with some visual and vibrotactile aids for the deaf. *American Annals of the Deaf*, 1968, *113*, 311–317.

Levin, S., & Erber, N.P. A vision screening program for deaf children. *The Volta Review*, 1976, *78*, 90–99.

Ling, D. Implications of hearing aid amplification below 300 CPS. *The Volta Review*, 1964, *66*, 723–729.

Ling, D. Three experiments in frequency transposition. *American Annals of the Deaf*, 1968, *113*, 283–294.

Ling, D. *Speech and the hearing-impaired child: Theory and practice*. Washington, DC: A.G. Bell Association for the Deaf, 1976.

Ling, D., & Doehring, D.G. Learning limits of deaf children for coded speech. *Journal of Speech and Hearing Research*, 1969, *12*, 83–94.

Ling, D., & Ling. A.H. *Aural habilitation*. Washington, DC: A.G. Bell Association for the Deaf, 1978.

Lowell, E.L., & Stoner, M. *Play it by ear*. Los Angeles: John Tracy Clinic, 1960.

Martin, L.F.A., Tong, Y.C., & Clark, G.M. A multiple-channel cochlear implant. *Archives of Otolaryngology*, 1981, *107*, 157–159.

Martony, J. On the correction of the voice pitch level for severely hard of hearing subjects. *American Annals of the Deaf*, 1968, *113*,195–202.

McLeod, R., & Guenther, M. Use of an ordinary telephone by an oral deaf person: A case history. *The Volta Review*, 1977, *79*, 435–442.

Merklein, R.A. A short speech perception test of severely and profoundly deaf children. *The Volta Review*, 1981, *83*, 36–45.

Miller, G.A. The perception of speech. In M. Halle(Ed.), *For Roman Jakobson*. the Hague: Mouton and Co., 1956.

Miller, G.A., & Nicely, P.E. An analysis of perceptual confusions among some English consonants. *Journal of the Acoustical Society of America*, 1955, *27*, 338–352.

Monsen, R.B. Toward measuring how well hearing-impaired children speak. *Journal of Speech and Hearing Research*, 1978, *21*, 197–219.

Monsen, R.B., & Shaughnessy, D.H. Improvement in vowel articulation of deaf children. *Journal of Communication Disorders*, 1978, *11*, 417–424.

Moog, J.S. Approaches to teaching pre-primary hearing-impaired children. *AOEHI Bulletin: Education of the Hearing Impaired*, (A.G. Bell Association for the Deaf), 1970, 53–59.

Moog, J.S. Language instruction determined by diagnostic observation. *The Volta Review*, 1975, *77*, 561–570.

Nickerson, R.S. Characteristics of the speech of deaf persons. *The Volta Review*, 1975, *77*, 342–362.

Nickerson, R.S., Kalikow, D.N., & Stevens, K.N. Computer-aided speech training for the deaf. *Journal of Speech and Hearing Disorders*, 1976, *41*, 120–132.

Nielsen, H.B., & Gilberg, I. Telephone performance of persons with hearing handicap in relation to speech reception threshold. *Scandinavian Audiology*, 1978, (Suppl. 8), 232–238.

Nober, E.H. Vibrotactile sensitivity of deaf children to high intensity sound. *Laryngoscope*, 1967, *77*, 2128–2146.

Northern, J.L., & Downs, M.P. *Hearing in children*. Baltimore: Williams & Wilkins, 1978.

Numbers, M.E., & Hudgins, C.V. Speech perception in present day education for deaf children. *The Volta Review*, 1948, *50*, 449–456.

Olsen, W.O. Acoustics and amplification in classrooms for the hearing-impaired. In F.H. Bess(Ed.), *Childhood deafness: Causation, assessment, and management*. New York: Grune & Stratton, 1977.

Osberger, M.J., & Danaher, E.M. Temporary conductive loss in students with severe sensorineural deafness. *The Volta Review*, 1974, *76*, 52–56.

Owens, E., Benedict, M., & Schubert, E.D. Consonant phonemic errors associated with pure-tone configurations and certain kinds of hearing impairment. *Journal of Speech and Hearing Research* 1972, *15*, 308–322.

Owens, E., & Telleen, C.C. Speech perception with hearing aids and cochlear implants. *Archives of Otolaryngology*, 1981, *107*, 160–163.

Pascoe, D.P. Frequency responses of hearing aids and their effect on the speech perception of hearing-impaired subjects. *Annals of Otology, Rhinology and Laryngology*, 1975, *84* (Suppl. 23), 1–40.

Pesonen, J. Phoneme communication of the deaf. *Annals of the Finnish Academy of Science*, 1968, *151* (Series B).

Peterson, G.E., & Barney, H.L. Control methods used in a study of the vowels. *Journal of the Acoustical Society of America*, 1952, *24*, 175–184.

Pflaster, G. Mirror, mirror on the wall. . . .? *Journal of Speech and Hearing Disorders*, 1979, *44*, 379–387.

Pickett, J.M. Speech-processing aids for communication handicaps: Some research problems. In D.B. Tower(Ed.), *The nervous system; Human communication and its disorders* (Vol. 3). New York: Raven Press, 1975.

Pickett, J.M., & Martin, E.S. Some comparative measurements of impaired discrimination for sound spectral differences. *American Annals of the Deaf*, 1968, *113*, 259–267.

Pickett, J.M., & Martony, J. Low-frequency vowel formant discrimination in hearing-impaired listeners. *Journal of Speech and Hearing Research*, 1970, *13*, 347–359.

Pickett, J.M., & Pickett, B.H. Communication of speech sounds by a tactual vocoder. *Journal of Speech and Hearing Research* , 1963, *6*, 207–222.

Pickett, J.M., Martin, E.S., Johnson, D., Smith, S.B., Daniel, Z., Willis, D., & Otis, W. On patterns of speech feature reception by deaf listeners. In G. Fant(Ed.), *Speech communication ability and profound deafness*. Washington, DC: A.G. Bell Association for the Deaf, 1972.

Pintner, R., Eisenson, J., & Stanton, M. *The psychology of the physically handicapped*. New York: F.S. Crofts, 1941.

Plant, G.L. The use of tactile supplements in the rehabilitation of the deafened: A case study *Australian Journal of Audiology*, 1979, *1*, 76–82.

Plomp, R. Auditory handicap of hearing impairment and the limited benefit of hearing aids. *Journal of the Acoustical Society of America*, 1978, *63*, 533–549.

Pollack, D. *Educational audiology for the limited hearing infant*. Springfield, IL: Charles C. Thomas, 1970.

Pollack, D. An acoupedic program. In C. Griffiths(Ed.), *Proceedings of the International Conference of Auditory Techniques*. Springfield, IL: Charles C. Thomas 1974.

Quick, M.A. A test for measuring achievement in speech perception among young deaf children. *The Volta Review*, 1953, *55* 28–31.

Risberg, A. Hearing capacity and speech sound perception. Paper presented at the International Symposium on Childhood Deafness. Mt. Pleasant, MI, 1976.

Risberg, A. Hearing loss and auditory capacity. Paper presented at Research Conference on Speech-Processing Aids for the Deaf, Gallaudet College, Washington, DC, 1977.

Risberg, A., Agelfors, E., & Boberg, G. Measurements of frequency-discrimination ability of severely and profoundly hearing-impaired children. *KTH Quarterly Progress Report*, 1975, (2–3), 40–48.

Risberg, A., & Spens, K.E. Teaching machine for training experiments on speech perception. *KTH Quarterly Progress Report*, 1967, (2–3), 72–75.

Romano, P.E., & Berlow, S. Vision requirements for lipreading. *American Annals of the Deaf*, 1974, *119*, 383–386.

Ross, M. Binaural versus monaural hearing aid amplification for hearing impaired individuals. In F.H. Bess(Ed.), *Childhood deafness*. New York: Grune & Stratton, 1977(a).

Ross, M. Classroom amplification. In W.R. Hodgson & P.H. Skinner(Eds.), *Hearing aid assessment and use in audiologic habilitation*. Baltimore: Williams & Wilkins, 1977(b).

Ross, M., Duffy, R.J., Cooker, H.S., & Sargeant, R.L. Contribution of the lower audible frequencies to the recognition of emotions. *American Annals of the Deaf*, 1973, *118*, 37–42.

Ross, M., Kessler, M.E., Phillips, M.E., & Lerman, J.W. Visual, auditory, and combined mode presentations of the WIPI test to hearing impaired children. *The Volta Review*, 1972, *74*, 90–96.

Ross, M., & Lerman, J.W. A picture identification test for hearing-impaired children. *Journal of Speech and Hearing Research*, 1970, *13*, 44–53.

Ross, M., & Tomassetti, C. Hearing aid selection for preverbal hearing-impaired children. In M.C. Pollack(Ed.), *Amplification for the hearing-impaired*. New York: Grune & Stratton, 1980.

Sanders, D.A. *Aural rehabilitation*. Englewood Cliffs, NJ: Prentice-Hall, 1971.

Schulte, K., The use of supplementary speech information in verbal communication. *The Volta Review*, 1978, *80*, 12–20.

Schwartz, J.R., & Black, J. W. Some effects of sentence structure on speechreading. *Central States Speech Journal*, 1967, *18*, 86–90.

Sher, A., & Owens, E. Consonant confusions associated with hearing loss above 2000 Hz. *Journal of Speech and Hearing Research*, 1974, *17*, 669–681.

Simmons, A.A. Content subjects through language. In H.G. Kopp(Ed.). *Curriculum: Cognition and content*. Washington, DC: A.G. Bell Association for the Deaf, 1968.

Simmons, A.A. Language and hearing. In L.E. Connor(Ed.), *Speech for the deaf child: Knowledge and use*. Washington, DC: A.G. Bell Association for the Deaf, 1971.

Sims, D.G. The validation of the CID Everyday Sentence Test for use with the severely hearing impaired. *Journal of the Academy of Rehabilitative Audiology*, 1975, *8*, 70–79.

Sims, D.G. Visual and auditory training for adults. In J. Katz(Ed.) *Handbook of clinical audiology* (2nd ed.). Baltimore: Williams & Wilkins, 1978.

Skinner, M. Speech intelligibility in noise-induced hearing loss: Effects of high-frequency compensation. *Journal of the Acoustical Society of America*, 1980, *67*, 306–317.

Smith, C.R. Hearing measures and speech intelligibility in deaf children. Paper presented at the Annual Convention of the American Speech-Language-Hearing Association, Chicago, IL, 1971.

Smith, C.R. Residual hearing and speech production in deaf children. *Journal of Speech and Hearing Research* , 1975, *18*, 795–811.

Sparks, D.W., Ardell, L.A., Bourgeois, M., Wiedmer, B., & Kuhl, P.K. Investigating the MESA (Multipoint Electrotactile Speech Aid); The transmission of connected discourse. *Journal of the Acoustical Society of America*, 1979, *65*, 810–815.

Speaks, C., Parker, B., Harris, C., & Kuhl, P. Intelligibility of connected discourse. *Journal of Speech and Hearing Research*, 1972. *15*, 590–602.

Stevens, K.N., Nickerson, R.S., Boothroyd, A., & Rollins, A.M. Assessment of nasalization in the speech of deaf children. *Journal of Speech and Hearing Research*, 1976, *19*, 393–416.

Sung, R.J., Sung, G.S., & Hodgson, W.R. A comparative study of physical characteristics of hearing aids on microphone and telecoil inputs. *Audiology*, 1974, *13*, 78–89.

Thornton, N.E., & Erber, N.P. Auditory-visual speech perception by hearing-impaired children. *Hearing Aid Journal*, 1979, *32*,(6), 32–33.

Trammell, J.L., & Owens, S.L. The test of auditory comprehension (TAC). Paper presented at the Annual Convention of the American Speech-Language-Hearing Association, Chicago, IL, 1977.

Urbantschitsch, V. *Über Hörübungen bei Taubstummheit und bei Ertaubing im Späteren Lebenalter.* Vienna: Urban und Schwarzenberg, 1895.

van Uden, A. *A world of language for deaf children.* Rotterdam, The Netherlands: Rotterdam University Press, 1970.

Villchur, E. Signal processing. In M. Ross & T.G. Giolas(Eds.), *Auditory management of hearing-impaired children.* Baltimore: University Park Press, 1978.

Walden, B.E., & Montgomery A.A. Dimensions of consonant perception in normal and hearing-impaired listeners. *Journal of Speech and Hearing Research,* 1975, *18,* 444–455.

Walden, B.E., Prosek, R.A., Montgomery, A.A., Scherr, C.K., & Jones, C.J. Effects of training on the visual recognition of consonants. *Journal of Speech and Hearing Research,* 1977, *20,* 130–145.

Watson, T.J. Speech audiometry for children. In A.W.G. Ewing(Ed.), *Educational guidance and the deaf child.* Washington, DC: Volta Bureau, 1957.

Watson, T.J. The use of hearing aids by hearing-impaired pupils in ordinary schools. *The Volta Review.* 1964, *66,* 741–744; 787.

Wedenberg, E. Auditory training for deaf and hard of hearing children. *Acta Oto-Laryngologica,* 1951, *39,* (Suppl. 94).

Wedenberg, E. Auditory training of severely hard of hearing preschool children. *Acta Oto-Laryngologica,* 1954, *44,* (Suppl. 110).

Weichbrodt, M. Tactual compared with visual discrimination of consonantal qualities. *Journal of General Psychology,* 1932, *4,* 203–206.

Whetnall, E., & Fry, D.B. *The deaf child.* Springfield, IL: Charles C Thomas, 1964.

Wilcox, J., & Tobin, H. Linguistic performance of hard-of-hearing and normal-hearing children. *Journal of Speech and Hearing Research,* 1974, *17,* 286–293.

Willemain, T.R., & Lee, F.F. Tactile pitch feedback for deaf speakers. *The Volta Review,* 1971, *73,* 541–553.

Yanick, P., & Freifield, S.(Eds.). *The application of signal processing concepts to hearing aids.* New York: Grune and Stratton, 1978.

Zaliouck, A. A visual-tactile system of phonetical symbolization. *Journal of Speech and Hearing Disorders,* 1954, *19,* 190–207.

Zeiser, M.L., & Erber, N.P. Auditory/vibratory perception of syllabic structure in words by profoundly hearing-impaired children. *Journal of Speech and Hearing Research ,* 1977, *20,* 430–436.

index
of subjects